CHRISTIAN HAMMÄCHER

IMPLANTS AND DENTURES – A WORKING SCRIPT

 Bibliographic information from the German National Library
The German National Library lists this publication in the German National Bibliography; detailed bibliographic data are available on the Internet at http://dnb.dnb.de.

First published in German as „Implantate und Zahnersatz – ein Arbeitsskript“ © 2021 by teamwork media GmbH & Co. KG
1. Edition (German edition): ISBN 978-3-00-069028-0

English translation © 2025
ISBN (English edition): 978-3-96474-841-6

Text/Layout/Production: mgo fachverlage GmbH & Co. KG, business premises Schwabmünchen
Franz-Kleinhans-Straße 7, 86830 Schwabmünchen,
www.mgo-dental.de
Printer: Generál Nyomda Kft., H-6728 Szeged, Kollégiumi út 11/H

mgo dental

Introduction

Implant dentistry and implant prosthodontics have become an integral part of a modern reconstructive dental treatment concept. Implant prosthodontics particular, is now part of the standard range of treatments offered by most dental practices and dental laboratories. After initial professional contacts during medical school, this exciting and diverse field is usually explored in more depth during the curricular or postgraduate period, in the dental practice, clinic and laboratory, as well as through individual further training.

From single-tooth replacements in the esthetic zone to anchoring fixed or removable dentures in partially edentulous jaws and supporting removable or fixed suprastructures in edentulous jaws: the wide range of applications in implant dentistry and implant prosthodontics represents a significant enrichment of the prosthetic treatment spectrum. This requires specific knowledge to achieve predictable results and avoid treatment failures. In addition to a well-founded treatment plan, the focus is on choosing an adequate restorative material as well as a suitable technique and execution. Parameters such as individual periodontal risks, a prosthetically appropriate implant position, a favorable combination of implants with natural teeth, as well as conventional prosthetic, orthodontic, and endodontic alternatives should be considered when planning treatment. However, surgical, periodontal and prosthodontics measures cannot be strictly separated from one another. The combination of these disciplines, which is essential for the success of the treatment, becomes particularly apparent in the therapy of the esthetic zone. The present script therefore covers not only implant prosthodontics but also surgical and periodontal surgical aspects, since these should be included in treatment planning and patient education from the outset.

This book, "IMPLANTS AND DENTURES – A WORKING SCRIPT" provides a good and structured overview of the complex subject of implant prosthodontics in a compact form that nevertheless covers the key areas in depth. The combination of scientific principles, informative clinical images, exemplary, well-documented case- reports, as well as practical tips and advice on avoiding complications and failures, makes it a stimulating reference work for daily dental practice and also for dental laboratories. As mentioned by Christian Hammächer in the introduction, it incorporates the content of his lecture as part of the DGI curriculum, both structurally and thematically. Like a continuous lecture on implant prosthodontics, it answers basic and complex questions in the specialist area in an easy-to-understand and entertaining manner. An extensive bibliography for further reading supports readers in deepening their knowledge on the subject. In my view, this manual is suitable for interested students, colleagues as well as dental technicians who wish to deepen their knowledge in the clinical and technical aspects of implant dentistry and implant prosthodontics.

Enjoy the read!

Sincerely Daniel Edelhoff

Content

1.

The single-tooth implant in the esthetic zone

2.

Implant-prosthetic restoration of the partially edentulous jaw

3.

Implant-prosthetic restoration of the edentulous jaw

Introduction

The idea for this book occurred to me during the second revision and update of the script accompanying the DGI curriculum. The script for the module “Implants and Dentures” of the DGI/APW implant dentistry curriculum was first prepared in 2010 with the support of Dr. Hanne Thomé. It closely followed the lectures in the corresponding module.

Likewise, it is divided into three topics: implant-based therapy in the esthetic zone as well as implant-prosthetic restoration of the partially and fully edentulous jaw. In 2020, I then updated it extensively and rewrote it for the most part. This book was created on the basis of the script due to the very positive response from participants in the curriculum over the past few years and the motivation to produce an affordable workbook on treatment options in implant prosthodontics. Many of the involved technical principles are based on the teaching of Prof. Hubertus Spiekermann, in whose department I worked for eight years before setting up my own practice. My special thanks go to him as a great teacher and mentor.

In line with his treatment philosophy, surgery and prosthodontics are therefore not treated as separate entities in the following book either. In particular, the chapter on implant-based therapy in the esthetic zone touches on the topic of hard and soft tissue management at the implant - in some parts also in depth. In addition to each of the three chapters mentioned above, together with their numerous clinical illustrations, a corresponding case report is presented and documented step by step in detail. In addition to a conclusion, practical tips on avoiding mistakes and on crisis management conclude the topic sections.

The book is intended as a true workbook aimed at students, colleagues who are interested in or work in implant dentistry, as well as interested dental technicians. It aims to be quickly accessible, provide suggestions, give a practical professional overview and answer questions that arise in day-to-day practical work, particularly with regard to the appropriate therapeutic approach for each individual. It is not intended as a replacement for a textbook in the traditional sense, but rather to spark interest in delving deeper into the subject matter.

At the end of this brief introduction, I would like to thank my co-practitioner in the clinic Prof. Jamal M. Stein: numerous interdisciplinary treatment approaches developed over the past few years have been incorporated into the book. In addition to our treatment team, I would also like to thank the dental laboratories Impladent, Alscher Dental and Van Iperen Zahntechnik for their dental work and excellent cooperation. Numerous dental photos, in particular by MDTs Volker Weber and Ralf Ommerborn, complement the script.

I would like to thank Ingrid Strobel (Camlog) for her positive suggestions in getting the project off the ground, and Dr. Alina Ion and Sigrid Eisenlauer (teamwork media Verlag) for their devoted and competent editorial and graphic implementation. I was particularly honored by the kind foreword by Prof. Daniel Edelhoff.

I hope you enjoy reading and working with the "script"!

Sincerely
Christian Hammächer

1

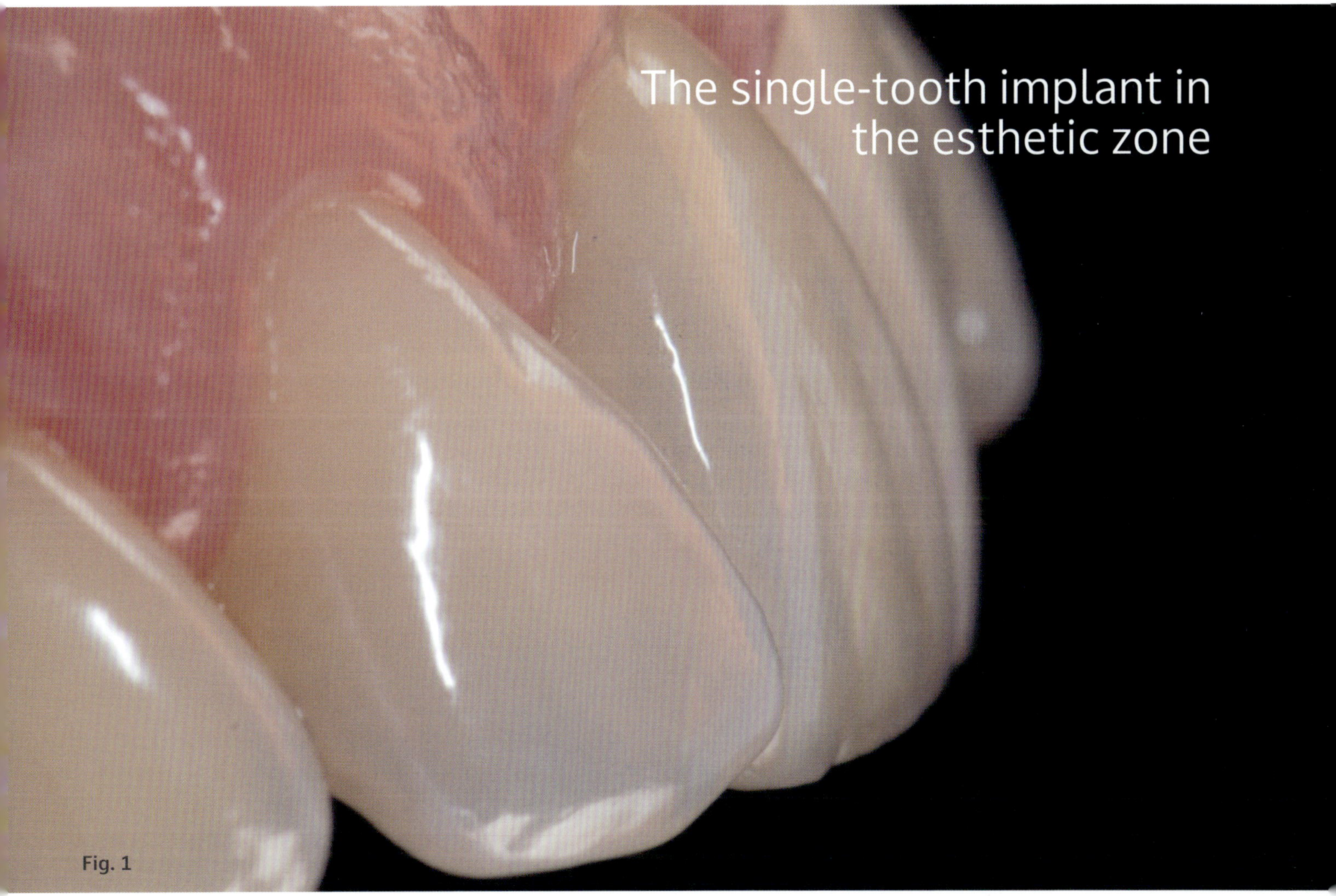

The single-tooth implant in the esthetic zone

Fig. 1

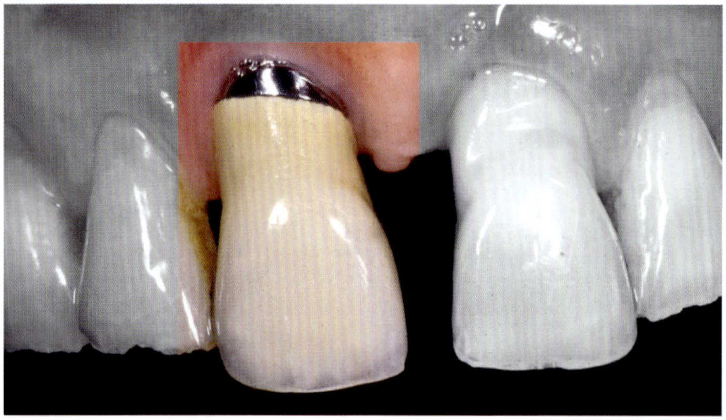

Fig. 2: Late-onset recession following flapless immediate implant placement of a periodontally compromised central incisor

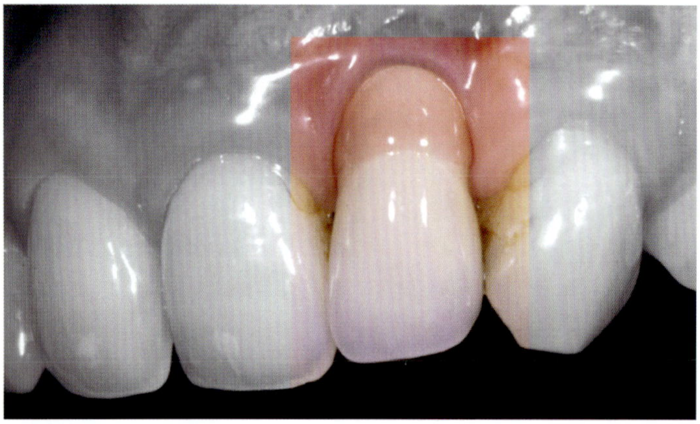

Fig. 3: Missing hard and soft tissue was replaced with pink ceramic.

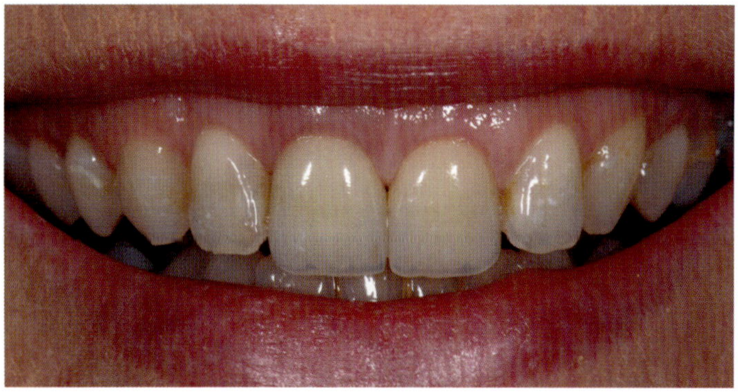

Fig. 4: Female patient with a high smile line

1.1.

Introduction

Of all the indications in endosseous implant dentistry, implant placement in the maxillary anterior region is certainly the most challenging.
This is especially true as the initial anatomical situation is rarely optimal and a natural-looking and esthetically pleasing end result for the patient depends crucially on the presence or absence of peri-implant hard and soft tissue (see previous page, Fig. **1**, single-tooth implant in region 11).
Prosthetic treatment options can help us to optimize the implant-prosthetic therapeutic approach. But do they also protect us from implant-prosthetic failures in the esthetic zone? The main parameters for successful implant therapy in the maxillary anterior region are a correct three-dimensional implant position as well as stable peri-implant hard and soft tissue. Disregarding these parameters is a compromise from the outset and may sooner or later lead to treatment failure, which can only be compensated to a limited extent with the implant-prosthetic therapy options available to us. (Figs. **2 & 3**).

1.2.

Analysis of the initial situation

At the beginning of every treatment plan, we discuss with the patient about their expectations and demands regarding the treatment outcome. During this discussion, the patient should also be informed about what results can be expected or are realistically achievable. In addition to the standard parameters of extra- and intraoral diagnostics, the contour of the smile line in the anterior tooth region requires special attention (Fig. **4**).

	"Thin" biotype	"Thick" biotype
Gingival thickness (Greenberg et al. 1976)	< 1.5 mm	≥ 1.5 mm
Scalloped contour (Seibert & Lindhe 1989)	high	flat
Transparency of the probe (Kan et al. 2010)	available	missing
Tooth shape (Olsson & Lindhe 1991) (Stein 2013)	triangular	square
(Olsson & Lindhe 1991) (Stein 2013)	triangular	square

Tab. 1

The focus of the intraoral examination is on the assessment of hard and soft tissue morphology. The respective "biotype" can be recognized by the thickness and quantity of the keratinized gingiva, as well as by the usually correlating parameters of gingival contour, papilla height and tooth shape. (Tab. 1) [1]. These anatomical conditions can prove crucial when deciding on the therapeutic approach. In principle, it is advisable for an esthetically long-term stable result to convert a thin biotype into a thick biotype during the course of therapy, if possible. [2]. The thick gingival type generally also appears to be associated with a rather thick buccal bone wall. [3]. In principle, attention should also be paid to any hard and soft tissue deficits (e.g. existing recessions), the gap width, the prognosis of the adjacent teeth as well as the overall esthetic appearance of the front.

1.3.

Treatment strategy

When considering implant placement in the esthetic zone, the following questions should be asked and the respective pros and cons weighed:

- Is the implant to be placed immediately after tooth extraction, in the sense of a delayed (immediate) implantat placement after six to eight weeks, or as a late implantat placement, possibly with preceding socket preservation measures?
- Is flap opening to be performed?
- Can a necessary hard-tissue augmentation be performed in one or two stages, and if so, how is it realized?
- Is healing intended subgingival or transgingival?
- When and how will prosthetic restoration take place?
- Should possibly necessary soft tissue optimization be performed immediately after extraction, as part of the implantat placement procedure, during re-entry or even before tooth extraction?

For each treatment case, it is important to determine the optimal individual treatment plan based on the given circumstances and to offer the patient the greatest possible degree of predictability.

Relevant success criteria in the esthetic zone

An esthetically pleasing final result with anterior implants depends on the following factors:

1. Hard and soft tissue situation/biotype
2. Correct three-dimensional implant alignment
   - Insertion angle
   - Insertion depth
   - Orovestibular alignment
   - Distance to adjacent teeth
3. Number of implants (for multiple implants)
4. Time of implantat placement
5. Dental technology
   - Abutment material/abutment fabrication
   - provisional/therapeutic/definitive restoration
6. Implant design
   - Implant geometry
   - Implant-abutment interface
   - Surface

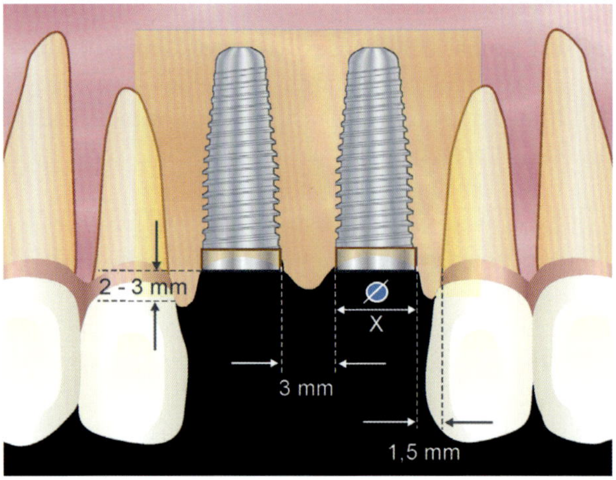

Fig. 5: Implant position in relation to the adjacent tooth or adjacent implant

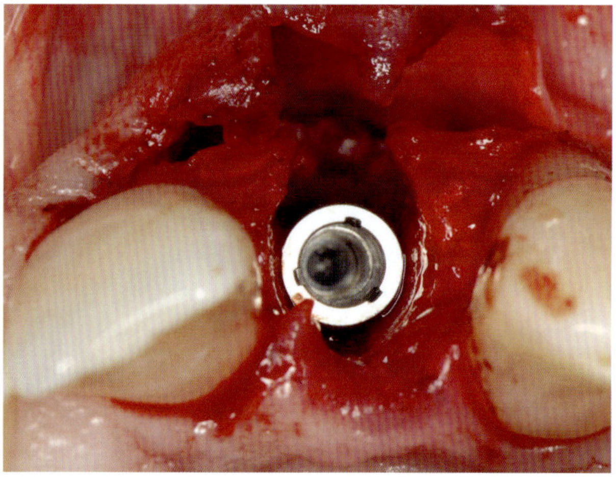

Fig. 6: Optimal implant position with vestibular incongruence defect

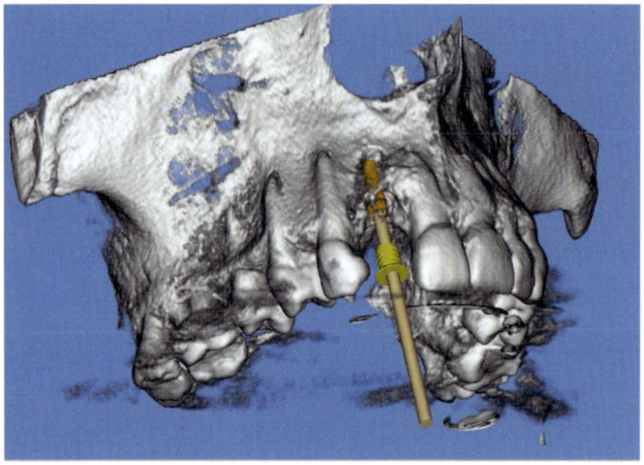

Fig. 7: Three-dimensional implant planning

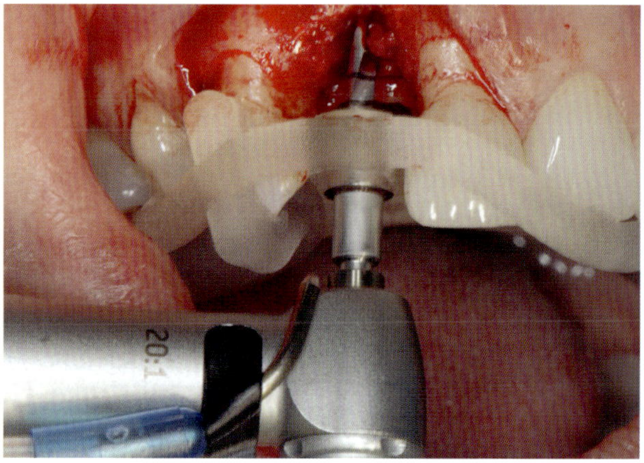

Fig. 8: Guided implant insertion using a surgical guide

1.4.

Implant position

The decisive factor for an esthetically satisfactory final outcome in the anterior region is the correct three- dimensional alignment of the implant, in addition to the peri-implant hard and soft tissue. This is determined by the angle and depth of insertion, the distance to the adjacent teeth as well as the orovestibular positioning (Figs. **5 & 6**). Three-dimensional implant planning based on prosthetic specifications can prove helpful in this context. (Figs. **7 & 8**).

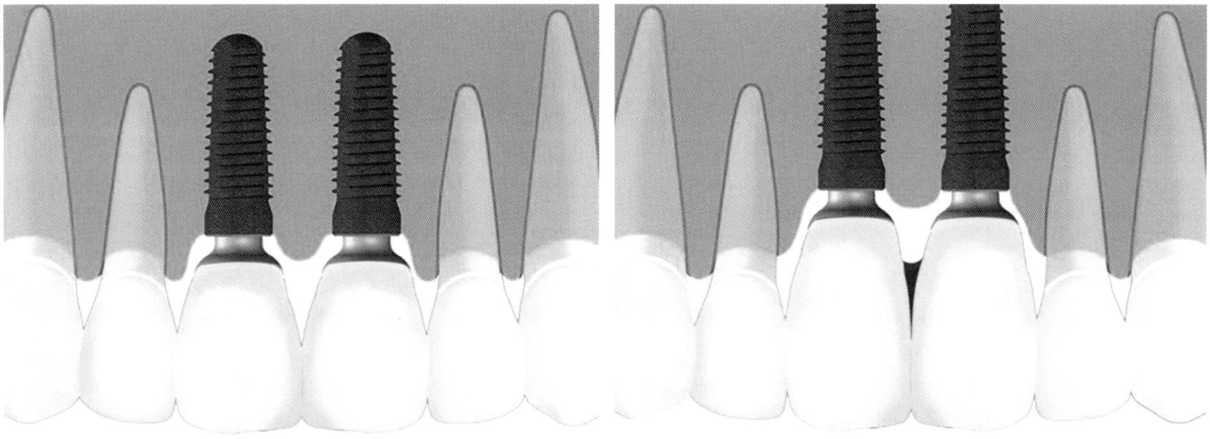

Figs. 9 a & b: Effects of the vertical implant position on crown length

The minimum distance between two implants should be 3 mm [4] and the distance to the tooth should not be less than 1.5 mm. If these distances are not taken into account, the presence of esthetically and functionally satisfactory interdental papillae can not be assumed. In the vertical dimension, the positioning of the implant shoulder is not primarily based on the existing bone level, but rather on the enamel cementum junction of the adjacent teeth in a healthy periodontium. As a rule, the implant shoulder should be located approx. 2-3 mm apically from the biological width (supracrestal tissue attachment), depending on its variation. Implants with "platform switching" can tend to be inserted somewhat deeper. If the specified distance to the enamel-cement border is exceeded, correspondingly long or longer crowns must be anticipated (Figs. **9a & b**).

For bucco-oral alignment, it can prove helpful, as described by C. Cacaci, to mentally or actually stretch a ligature around the adjacent teeth and to ensure that the distance to the buccal cord remains as large as possible. Particular care must be taken to the palatal alignment of the implant in the socket, especially in the case of immediate implant placement. The prerequisite for this is a primary drilling that is significantly further palatal than the former root or its apex in its axis and alignment. If the implants tend towards being anchored palatally in the extraction socket, the risk of recession formation at the connection is less than with implants placed more facially. When placing the implant, there is often a tendency of drifting vestibularly (especially with the last turns and at high primary stability), which is partly due to the tensile strength of the palatal compacta. The implant essentially selects the path of least resistance. This effect is more pronounced if the implant is not sufficiently anchored outside the alveolus and in root- shaped implants, and can lead to malpositioning with consecutive resorption of the buccal bone lamella and the risk of late dehiscence. Undesired buccal positioning of the implant and the associated disadvantages can be counteracted by palatal overcompensation of the pilot drilling. For this purpose, a "guide groove" is prepared on the palatal alveolar wall, as it were. Three-dimensional planning and implementation using a precision drilling template (system-inherent errors must be given particular consideration here [5]) can provide additional safety.

1.5.
Time of implant placement

The timing of implant placement and restoration of the socket after extraction also play an important role in the predictability of the treatment outcome. A section of the maxilla in the anterior region, in which an extraction socket is neither restored by early implant placement and augmentation or by socket preservation measures, will decrease in width by up to 50% and in vertical dimension by up to 2-4.5 mm within twelve months. This occurs mainly in the area of the buccal wall and then essentially in the first three months following tooth extraction [6]. After a year without the above-mentioned therapeutic interventions, such a situation is very difficult to reverse to an esthetically satisfactory result, especially in the presence of a high smile line. The extent of post- extraction bone resorption changes depending on the trauma to the alveolar walls, their thickness as well as the extent of pathological processes that influence bone regeneration both before and after extraction. In principle, it can be assumed here that the covering mucosa tends to follow the shape of the underlying bone. In particular, localized pathological processes apical or circumferential to the affected tooth root can damage the socket and thus lead to dehiscences.

These dehiscence defects bear the risk of disrupting full osseous regeneration [7]. Minor defects can, under certain circumstances, be augmented simultaneously with immediate implant placement using autogenous bone or bone substitute material. In the case of extensive defects, it is advisable to refrain from immediate implant placement to avoid long-term complications. In these situations implant placement should tendencially delayed following prior or simultaneous augmentation. A case-by-case decision must be made on how to deal with chronically infected, root-fractured, perforated or similarly compromised roots.

Even though the failure rate of immediate implant placement is slightly increased in teeth with chronic apical periodontitis [8], the overall survival rate does not appear to be significantly reduced compared to delayed implant placement in healed defects. It would appear that immediate implant placement can be successfully performed in the case of limited periapical infection after thorough curettage [9, 10]. Immediate implant placement should be avoided in cases of extensive or acute inflammation.

1.5.1.
Immediate implant placement

In general, it can be recommended that teeth be extracted before immediate implant placement using the least traumatic procedure possible. In this case, instruments such as the periotome (Fig. **10**) or special extraction devices with a purely axial direction of pull can prove helpful

Dislocation movements, especially in the bucco-oral direction, should be avoided here if possible. The aim

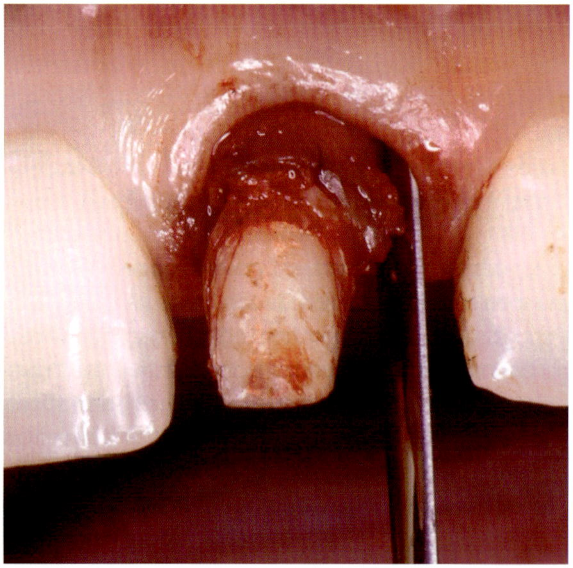

Fig. 10: Atraumatic tooth extraction using a periotome

of the procedure is to protect the often very thin buccal bone lamella and to preserve it as far as possible. Following extraction, the buccal bone wall should be checked for integrity by probing.

Immediate implant placement is usually not sufficient to prevent resorption of the buccal bone wall [11]. Even with flapless immediate implant placement, there is a vertical reduction in the buccal wall as well as in the width of the alveolar ridge. Although this is somewhat less pronounced than during implant insertion using flap formation [12] due to the absence of deperiostomy , its intensity depends on the implant position, the thickness of the buccal wall as well as the soft tissue. Despite the advantages of the flapless procedure [13], the author's recommendation, especially for surgeons with little clinical experience, is to visualize the implant placement site by means of a flap, to gain an overview of the bony situation and thus ensure the correct implant position. (Figs. **11 a & b**).

As a rule, a loss of vestibular gingival height must be expected with almost every immediate implant placement if appropriate compensatory measures are not taken or if a thick buccal bone wall is present. Significant recessions occur mainly when the implant is positioned too far buccally and the soft tissue type is thin [14, 15].

An interesting alternative therapeutic procedure is the so-called “socket shield technique” [16]. In combination with immediate implantplacement, a generally labial part of the tooth root is deliberately left in place here to prevent the bundle bone or buccal wall from being resorbed due to the extraction. (Fig. **12**). This procedure may be indicated in particular for very thin buccal walls or ankylosed teeth where a greater extraction trauma is to be expected.

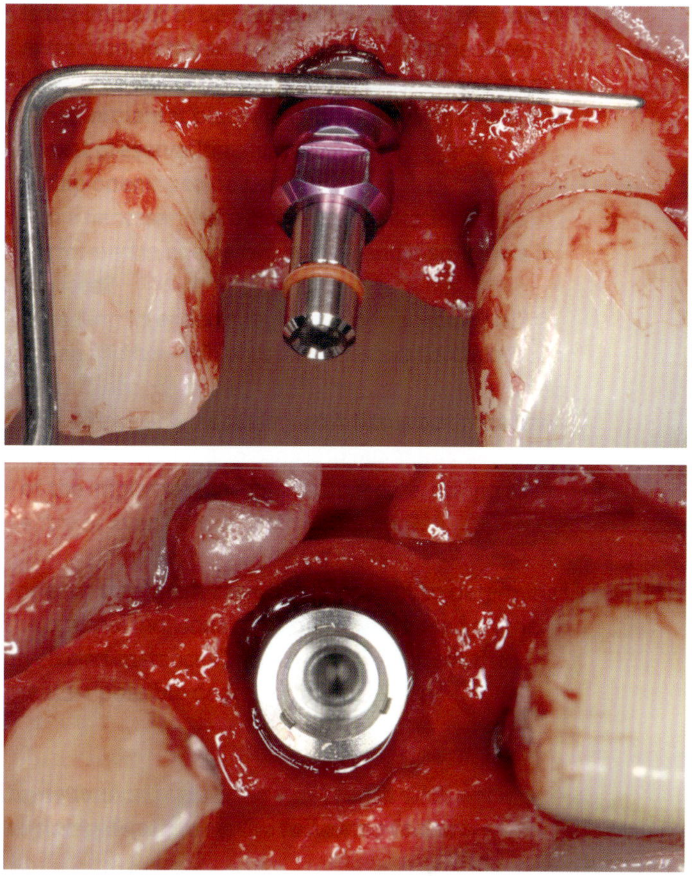

Figs. 11 a & b: Immediate implant placement while observing the correct three-dimensional implant position → aim for a palatal implant position!

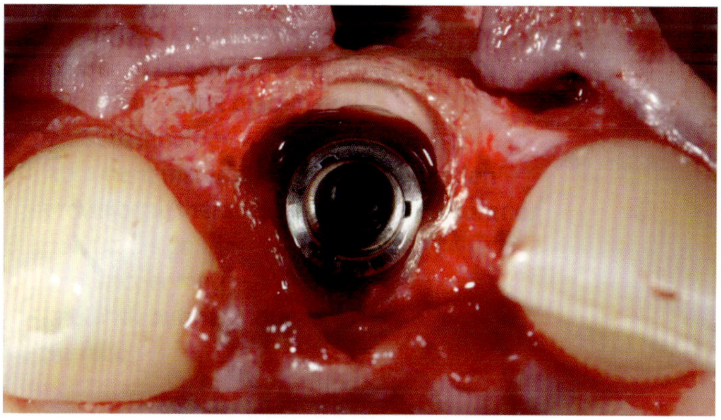

Fig. 12: "Socket shield technique": The labial root portion of the tooth, which in this case was ankylosed, was left in place.

There are different opinions on how to deal with incongruity defects, which almost always occur due to the mostly oval morphology of the extraction socket: in the case of defects where the distance between the implant surface and the socket wall is less than 2 mm, there is a high probability of spontaneous bone regeneration [17]. The surface characteristics of implants also have an additional influence if the incongruity defect is not filled. For example, a rough surface has a positive effect on bone regeneration as it promotes stabilization of the coagulum. A study by Botticelli et al. showed that defects of up to 3 mm in size could heal without augmentation by stabilizing the blood clot in the presence of a rough implant surface [18].

As already mentioned, the buccal bone lamella is also subject to resorption processes when an implant is inserted immediately. In an animal study on bone regeneration following immediate implant placement, Araujo et al. found that there was no difference in the resorption of the buccal bone wall after three months with regard to the placement of an implant in the fresh extraction socket or not. In all study groups, there was a reduction of at least 2 mm in vertical bone height.

However, filling the defect with a bone substitute material appears to reduce the resorption processes in the buccal wall [19]. This appears logical in view of the results of socket preservation. For appropriately large incongruence defects, the author therefore recommends filling with autologous bone chips or bone substitute material.
In the case of "standard incongruity defects", there is no need to use a membrane as this relates to a self- stabilizing multi-wall defect. Larger hard tissue defects (Figs. **13 a & b**) must be augmented and, if necessary, covered with a membrane within the context of the GBR technique. No standardized recommendation can be given for augmentation materials and techniques. However, when using membranes, the author generally prefers absorbable products because they reduce the likelihood of membrane exposure and wound dehiscence.

The decision to proceed with immediate implant placement must be made diligently in every case. The presence of inflammation, an "untreated" thin gingival type, as well as a weak palatal bone wall, possibly with an hourglass-shaped cross-section (in which case primary drilling cannot be safely positioned palatally), mean that immediate implant placement is not recommended.

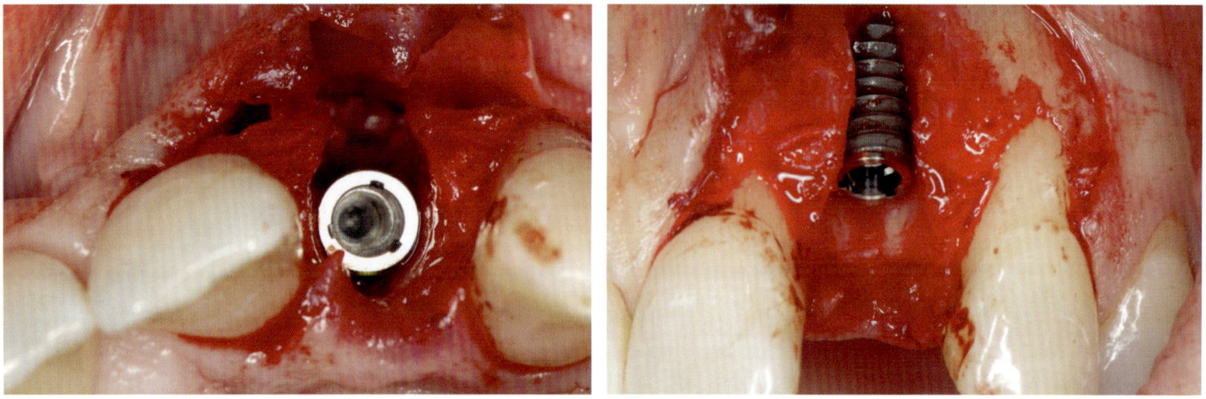

Figs. 13 a & b: Immediate implant placement in the case of a pronounced hard tissue defect in the area of the buccal wall

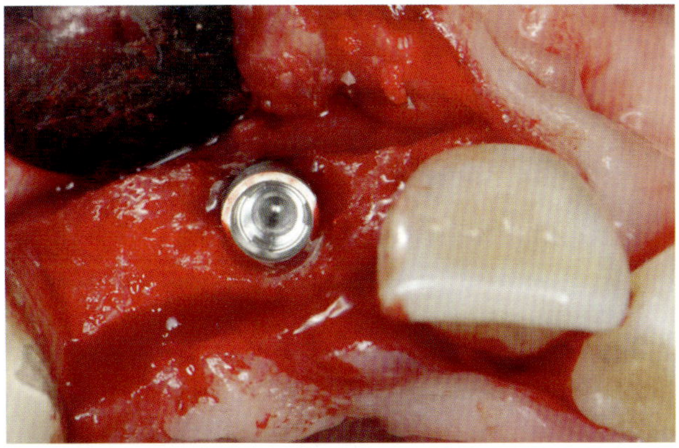

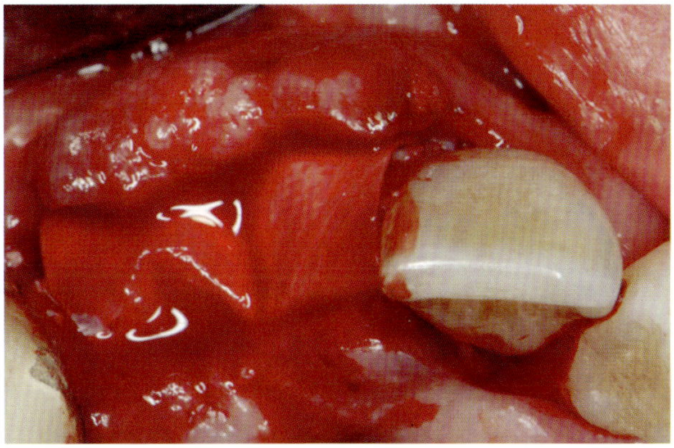

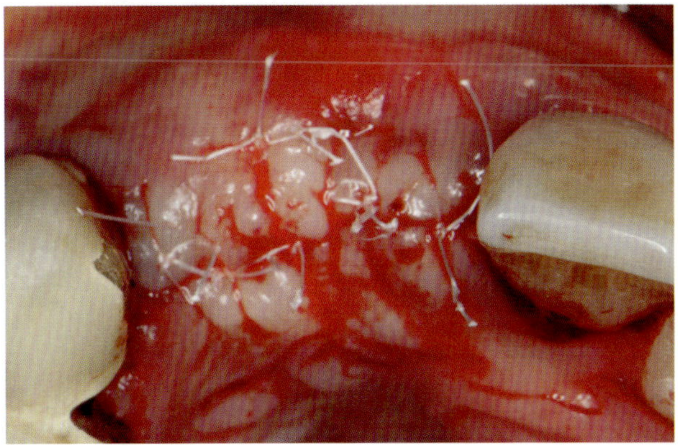

Figs. 14 a – c: Delayed implant placement with simultaneous augmentation using GBR with autologous bone, xenogeneic bone substitute and ribose cross-linked resorbable collagen membrane

In such cases, delayed or late implant placement is to be preferred, which, in conjunction with augmentative or soft tissue optimizing measures (socket preservation, socket seal techniques, e.g. combined grafts) at different times, usually provides more predictable and long-term stable results.

1.5.2.
Delayed implant placement

With regard to the timing of implant placement, different procedures have been described in the literature, so that no uniform definition of the terms immediate, delayed and late implant placement can be given.

In delayed implant placement, the soft tissue defect heals in approximally six to eight weeks after extraction (classification according to Spiekermann 1994). Bone regeneration begins at the base of the defect and in the area of the alveolar walls, and a closed soft tissue cover is formed. This offers the advantage that a dense wound closure can be predictably achieved in the event of augmentation. The resulting soft tissue plug in the upper part of the socket can, under certain circumstances, be used to positively thicken the soft tissue and should therefore not be routinely excised. (Figs. **14 a – c**).

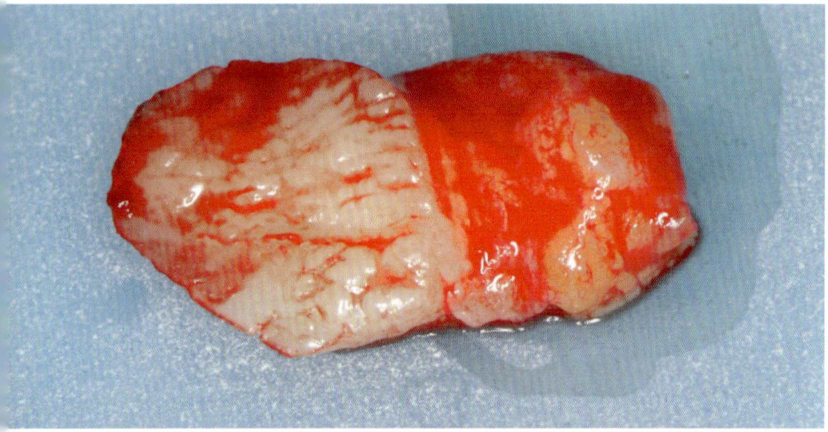

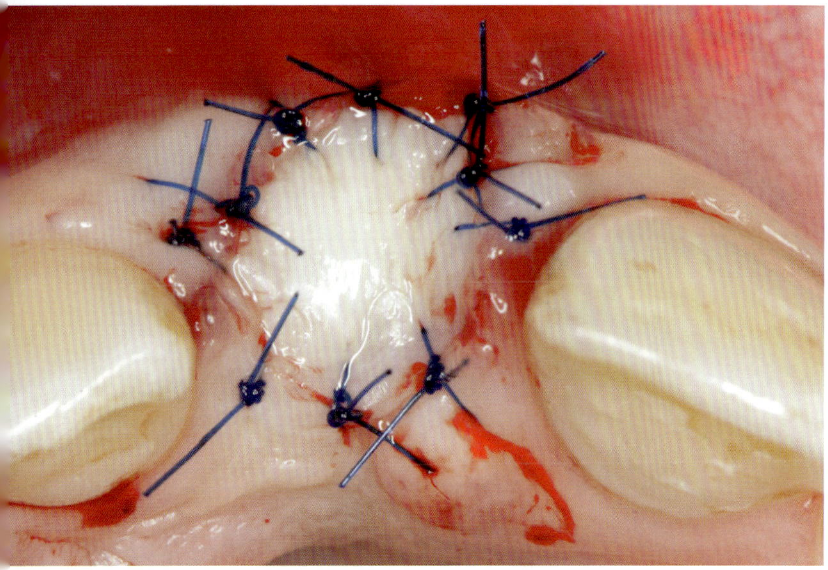

Figs. 15 a & b: combination transplant (FGG with connective tissue flap) from the palate

1.5.3.

Late implant placement and measures to maintain the alveolar ridge

Late implant placement refers to an implant placement four or more months after extraction. Implant placement is delayed until the socket has fully ossified and the soft tissue has completely healed (Spiekermann 1994).

Thus, a late implant placement also includes existing gaps that have been treated otherwise or not yet treated. In the case of a planned late implant placement, it may be advisable to consider ridge prophylaxis (socket preservation, ridge preservation, socket seal) within the context of extraction. The aim of these procedures and techniques is to protect the buccal bone lamella from resorption after extraction by introducing bone substitute material, collagen or autogenous bone into the socket, with the additional use of a membrane if the alveolar wall is not intact – to protect the buccal bone lamella from resorption after extraction, to stabilize the space and, if necessary, to optimize the soft tissue situation by means of different graft covers. However, additional covering of the bone substitute material in the area of the buccal wall does not appear to prevent further bony resorption [20].
This procedure is particularly indicated and useful in situations where tooth extraction or tooth loss has resulted in major hard and soft tissue defects due to inflammation, making prompt implant placement impossible. Histologically, however, one hardly gains more bone than with conventional alveolar healing [21], instead, the space is primarily preserved for later implant placement or augmentation, possibly combined with soft tissue optimizing measures (FGG, combination graft). It is important to note that the measures to maintain the ridge generally do not prevent a collapse in the volume of bone and are therefore not a substitute for later augmentation in numerous cases. Here, too, there is a correlation between the thickness of the buccal wall and the potential loss of volume: in a study by Cardaropoli [22], up to 85% of the initial dimension of the alveolar ridge could be maintained by socket preservation with bone substitute material and collagen membrane, regardless of the thickness of the buccal wall. In contrast, the study by Spinato [23] showed that the volume shrinkage after socket seal techniques was indeed dependent on the thickness of the buccal wall. This result seemingly contradicts the results

of Cardaropoli. On closer inspection, his results can be explained by the fact that, with the exception of one front tooth, only premolars and molars were examined, which usually have a significantly thicker buccal wall.

In the ridge-preserving procedures after extraction, the socket is covered with resorbable collagen matrices, thick FGGs from the palate or tuber, or combined soft tissue grafts (CTG plus FGG). (Figs. **15 a & b**). In addition to the procedure described by Stimmelmayr [24] for the palatally and vestibularly swung connective tissue portion, the modified socket seal technique published by Stein and Hammächer [25] (see Fig. **19**) involves the connective tissue portion being introduced approximal after tunneling the adjacent papillae.

The objective of all these techniques is to prevent resorption, maintain space as well as to optimize soft tissue. For filling the socket, the use of a slowly resorbing material is generally recommended, especially for prosthetic ridge augmentation. Even a thin gingival type can be transformed into a thick biotype by means of ridge prophylaxis in combination with soft tissue optimizing measures. The effort for the ridge-preserving measures should be evaluated individually and depends on the initial situation before extraction, according to the overview in the Figures **16 to 18**.
For the sake of completeness, the option of closing the socket after tooth extraction with root segments (TMC concept according to Neumeyer) should also be mentioned. The prerequisite for good integration of these segments is a preserved periodontium.

Overview of socket-seal techniques

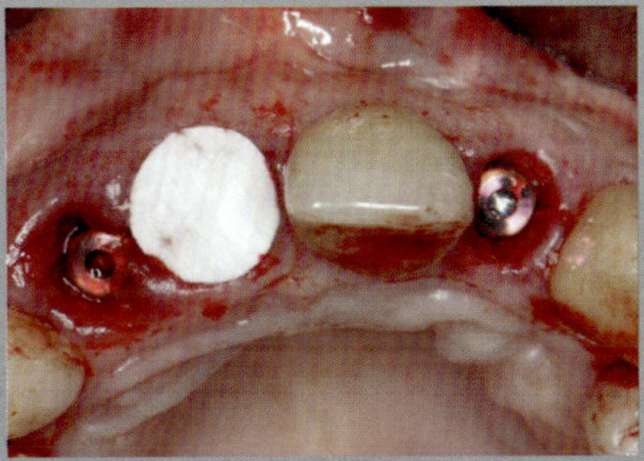

Socket-seal technique with a collagen matrix (Fig. 16)

- Thick gingiva type
- High esthetic standards
- No lack of buccal volume/thick biotype/thick buccal wall

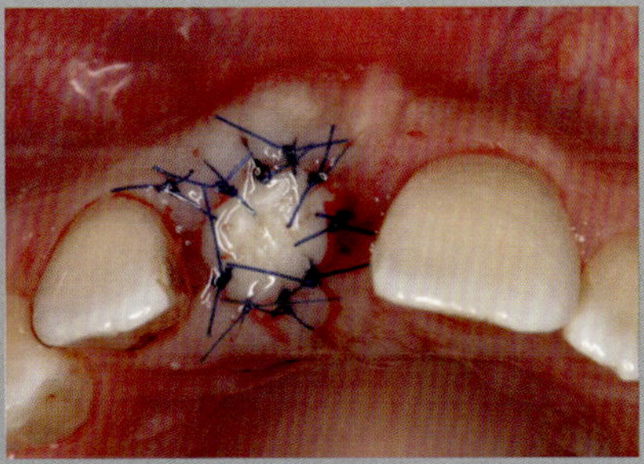

Simplified socket seal technique (FGG punch) (Fig. 17)

- Thin gingiva type
- High esthetic standards
- No lack of buccal volume

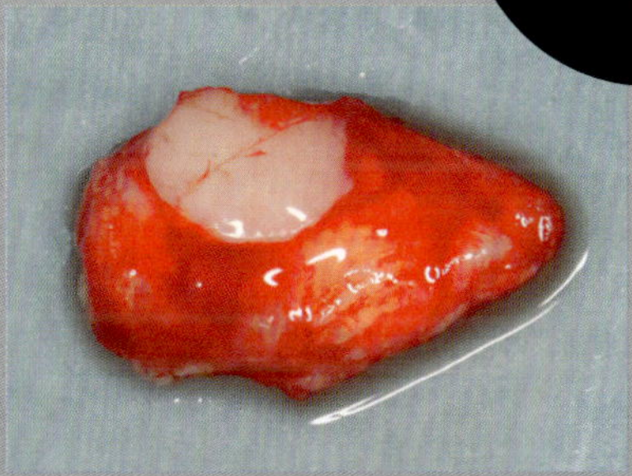

Modified socket seal technique (combination graft) (Fig. 18)

- Thin gingiva type
- Highest esthetic standards
- Lack of buccal volume

Figs. 19 a – i: Modified socket seal technique [25] (Stein/ Hammächer

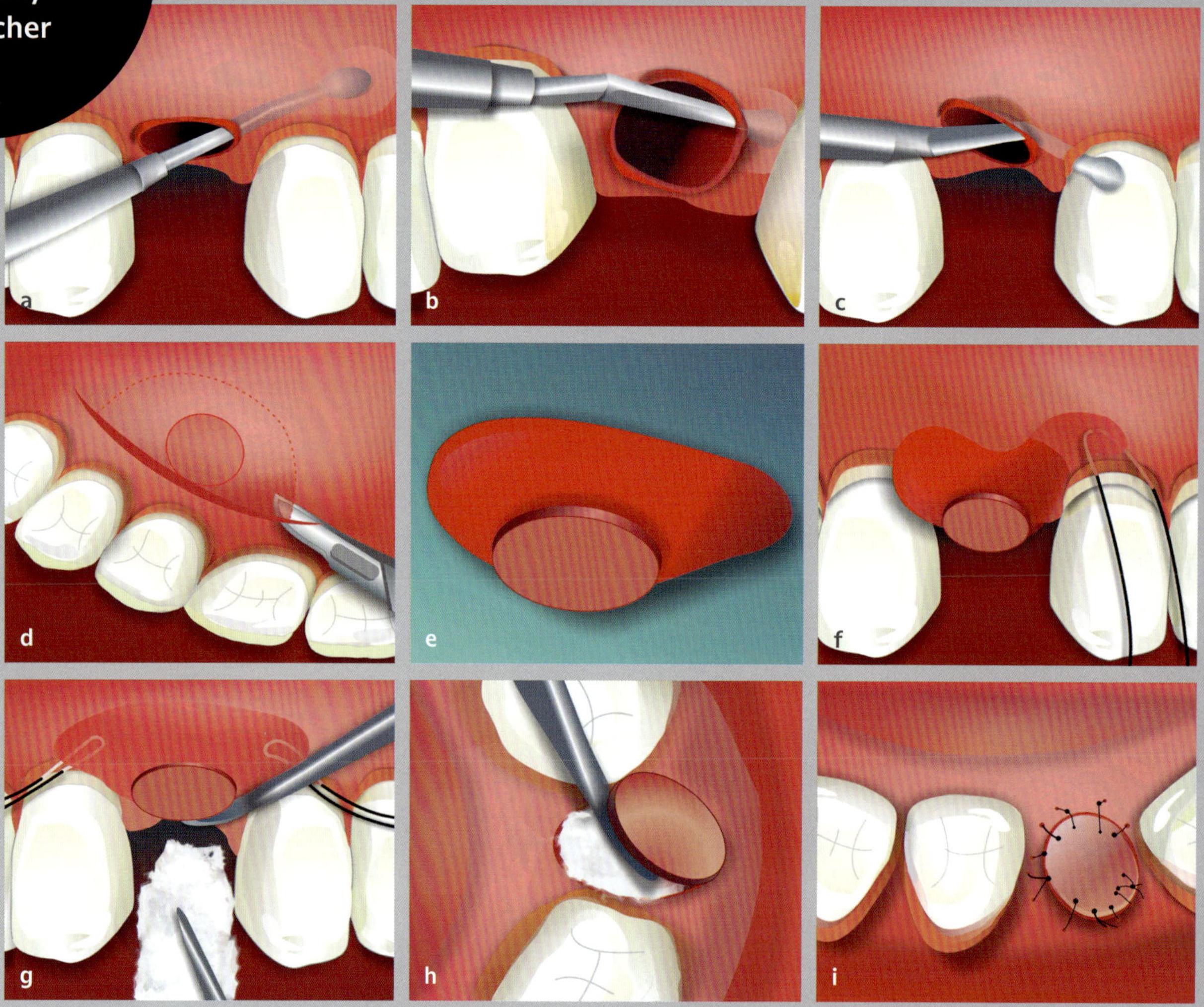

a – c) Tunneling of the vestibular gingival portions including the papillae adjacent to the extraction socket
d – e) Harvesting of a special combination transplant (FGG with a tendency towards laterally protruding CTG sections) from the palate
f) Insertion of the CTG portions into the prepared tunnel, whereby the connective tissue lies vestibularly and also under the papillae.
g) Filling of the socket with a slowly resorbing bone substitute material
h) Closure of the socket with the FGG
i) Fixation with single button sutures and cross-mattress sutures

[25] Stein JM, Hammächer C: Postextraction Socket Seal Surgery with an Epithelized Connective Tissue Graft using a Subpapillar Tunneling Procedure. Int J Periodontics Restorative Dent 2015; 35: 877–884

1.6.

Alternative strategies for soft tissue optimization and conditioning

If tooth extraction can still be planned, one of our favorite procedures is to **thicken the soft tissue using a modified tunnel technique prior to extraction** (Figs. **20 a & b, 21 a & b).** According to recession coverage in the tunnel technique on the natural tooth, this can be performed predictably [26, 27]. Furthermore, the buccal bone wall is still supported and is restored via the periodontal gap.

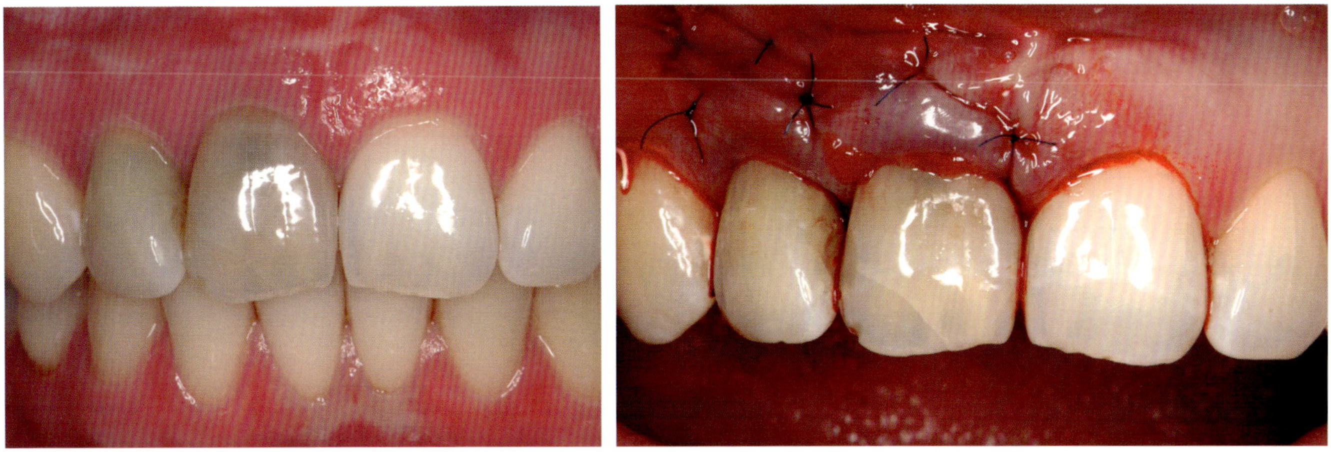

Figs. 20 a & b: Soft tissue thickening using a modified tunnel technique and CTG prior to planned tooth extraction of 11

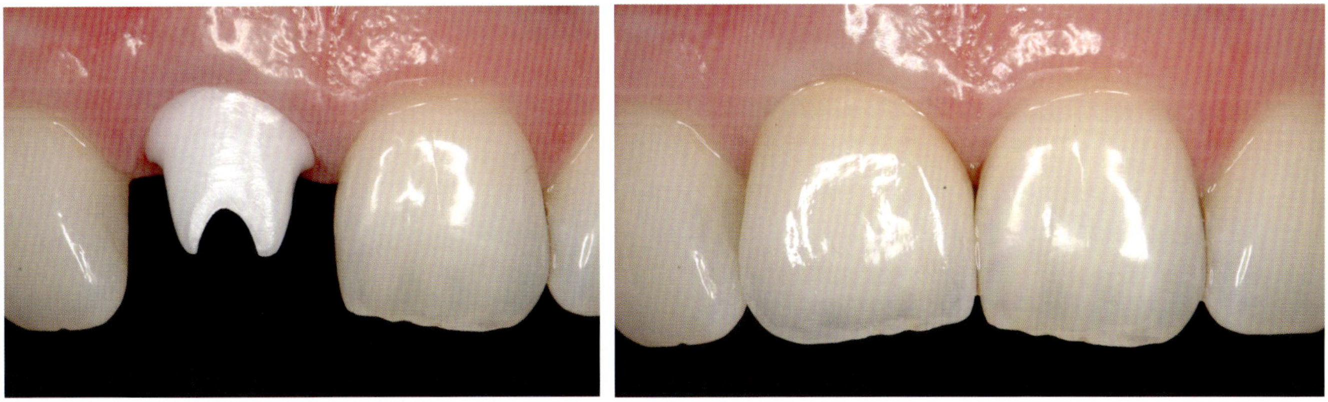

Figs. 21 a & b: Immediate implant placement with flap elevation after three months, immediate restoration and final resoration with individualized CAD/CAM zirconia hybidabutment and cemented crown

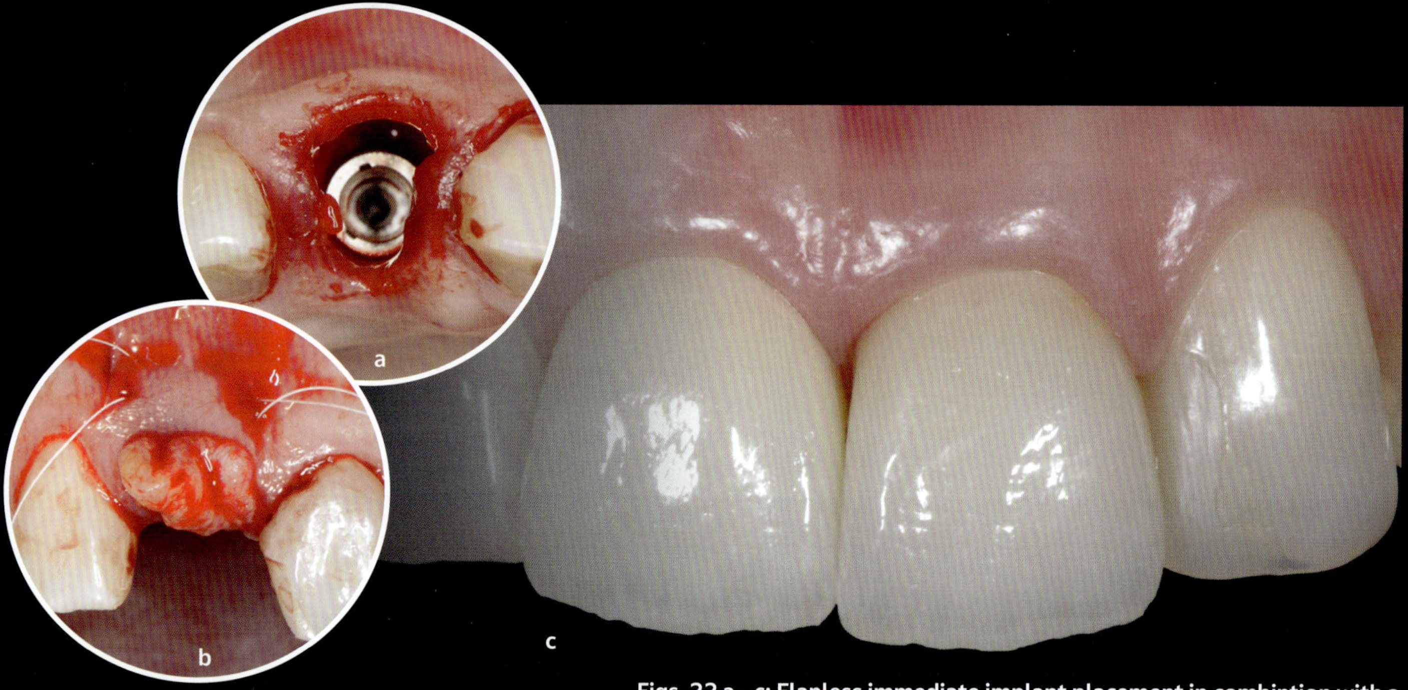

Figs. 22 a – c: Flapless immediate implant placement in combintion with a simultaneous CTG. Restoration using a screw-retained hybrid crown.

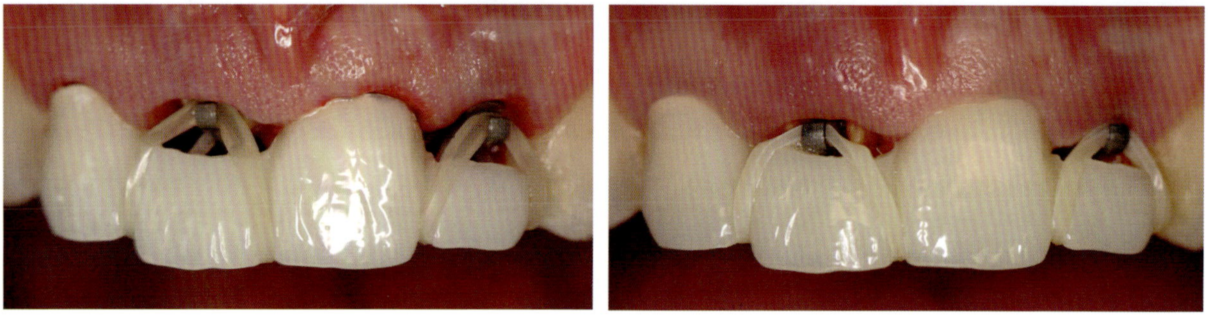

Figs. 23 a & b (image: J. M. Stein): Forced extrusion as a pre-implant measure for tissue conditioning according to the "TMC concept"

Simultaneously with immediate implant placement, connective tissue grafts can be used to thicken the vestibular gingiva, possibly using the tunnel technique (Figs. **22 a – c**). Care should be exercised here to ensure that the thin buccal wall is not traumatized during tunneling.

Conditioning of hard and soft tissue via extrusion
Extrusion or forced extrusion ("TMC concept" according to Neumeyer) can achieve vertical optimizations in terms of hard and soft tissue (Figs. **23 a & b**), and this entirely without the use of substitute materials according to corresponding biological concepts. These procedures can thus be employed as a sensible and gentle pre-implant therapy option.

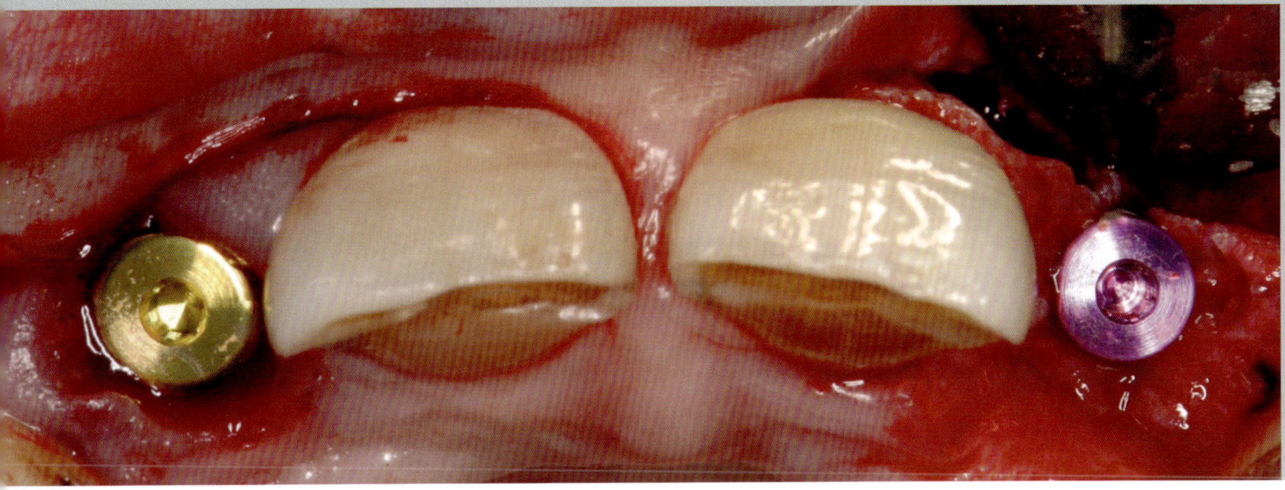

Fig. 24: immediate implant placement in region 12 and delayed implant placement in region 22

1

1.7.

Comparison of immediate implant placement, delayed implant placement and late implant placement

When comparing the different procedures, the following can be concluded: in terms of implant survival rates, the literature does not show any significant difference between delayed and immediate implant placement in the anterior tooth region (Fig. **24**). For both procedures, loss rates of less than 5% have been reported [28, 29]. In terms of the final esthetic result, both immediate and delayed implant placement also appear to be virtually equivalent. However, Chen reports of a greater risk of recession with immediate implant placement in his review [30]. Block et al. [31] compared the hard and soft tissue response in the maxillary anterior tooth region for immediate implant placement with immediate restoration versus late implant placement (four months after socket preservation). They observed no significant difference in terms of bone loss, but the immediate implant placement group demonstrated an average of one millimeter more vestibular gingiva. In a review article, Hartog et al. [32] also examined the different procedures (immediate implant placement , delayed implant placement and late implant placement) with regard to hard and soft tissue progression, patient satisfaction and esthetics. Overall, there were no significant differences in survival rate and peri-implant bone loss when comparing immediate implant placement, delayed implant placement, and late implant placement

In conclusion, it can be stated that all the described procedures can lead to satisfactory results, if the indication and the procedure in the esthetic zone are managed correctly. The respective initial situation is crucial and determines the individually appropriate therapeutic approach to be adopted. As shown in the previous chapters, this can be as diverse in the esthetic zone as in no other indication area in implant dentistry.

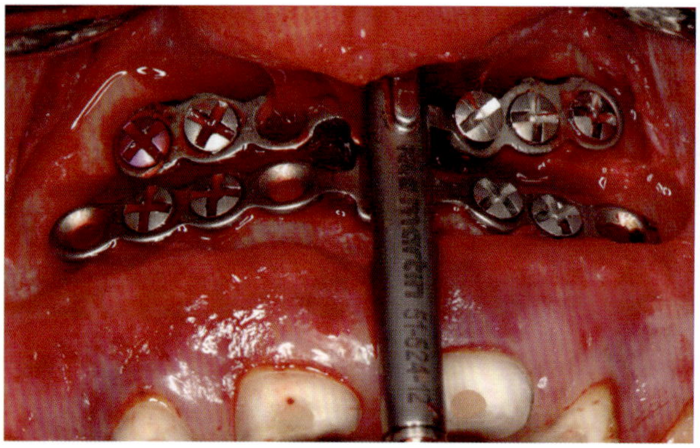

Fig. 25: Distraction osteogenesis in the anterior maxilla region

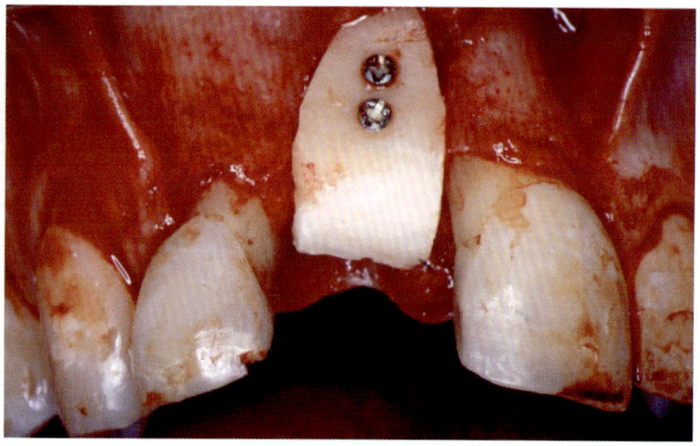

Fig. 26: "J-graft“ from the mandibular angle for augmentation in region 11

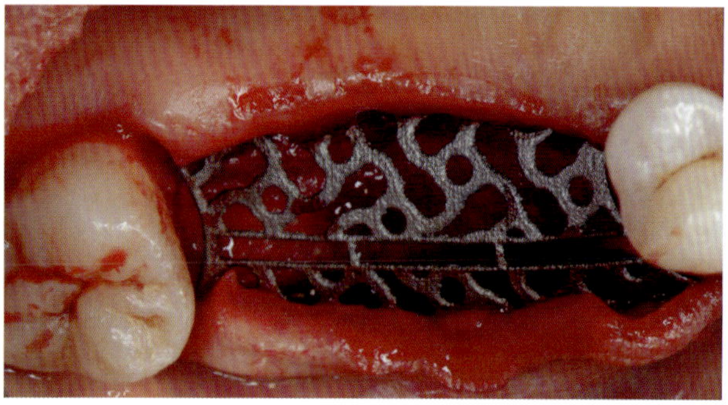

Fig. 27: Customized titanium mesh for vertical and lateral augmentation in the posterior maxilla region

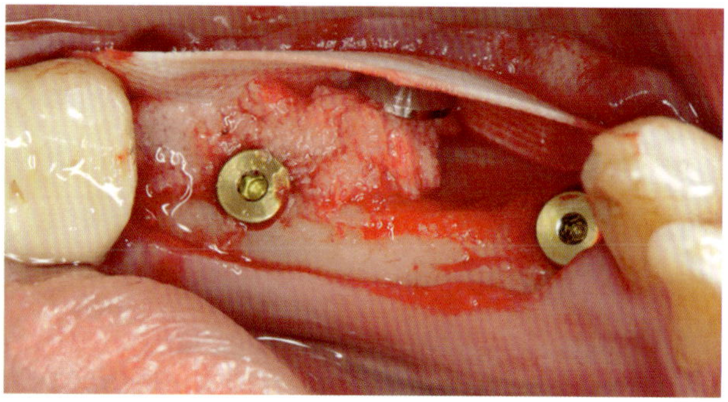

Fig. 28: GBR with support screw in the posterior mandibular region

Overall, parameters such as the esthetics of the final result, the gingival situation as well as patient satisfaction are clearly underrepresented in the literature. In most older publications, implantological success was assessed solely on the basis of the implant survival rate in terms of osseointegration.
It is not possible to give a clear assessment of which technique is superior in terms of predictability and stability of the final esthetic result. Of course, it is also important here to note the initial anatomical situation at the start of the respective therapy and that not every surgical technique leads to the same results in different hands.

1.8.

Augmentation techniques

The recession of hard and soft tissue presents a major challenge for the clinician, especially in patients with a high smile line. Here, various augmentation procedures can be used to rebuild lost bone. If a tissue deficit is detected, it should first be decided, possibly using a digital volume tomography in combination with an examination of the clinical situation, whether augmentation can or must be performed simultaneously or in two stages.

In our treatments, simultaneous augmentation usually involves the use of GBR. Resorbable collagen membranes, shells with different resorption times, non-resorbable membranes or even individually milled titanium meshes (Fig. **27**) cover and stabilize particulate autologous bone (Fig. **26**) or different bone graft materials. The use of PRF (platelet-rich fibrin) can have a positive effect on the healing process.
In the two-stage procedure, and depending on the defect morphology, augmentation can be performed using GBR, autologous or allogeneic bone blocks or autologous, allogenic and synthetic bone shells. (Fig. **28**). With the so-called "tentpole technique", a vertical structure can even be achieved in small gaps using GBR. For larger segments and non-restricted bone width, distraction osteogenesis (Fig. **25**) is particularly suitable for vertical augmentation.
The decision for the respective procedure depends on the size and shape of the defect. In the anterior tooth region, particular attention must be taken to maintaining the "soft tissue architecture" and to the subsequent esthetic expectations.

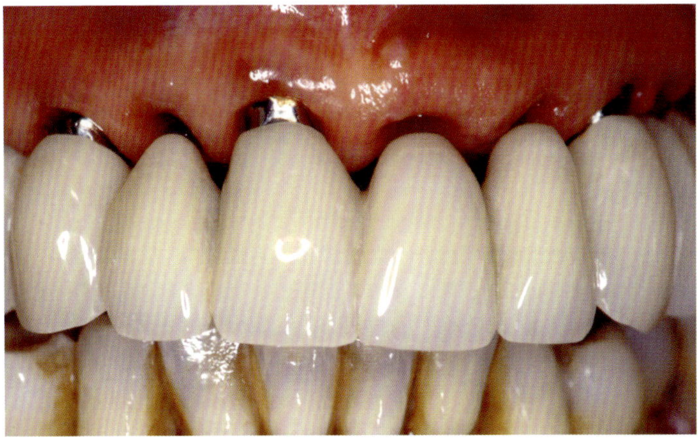

Fig. 29: Ovate pontics maintaining and creating papillae in a fixed provisonal restoration

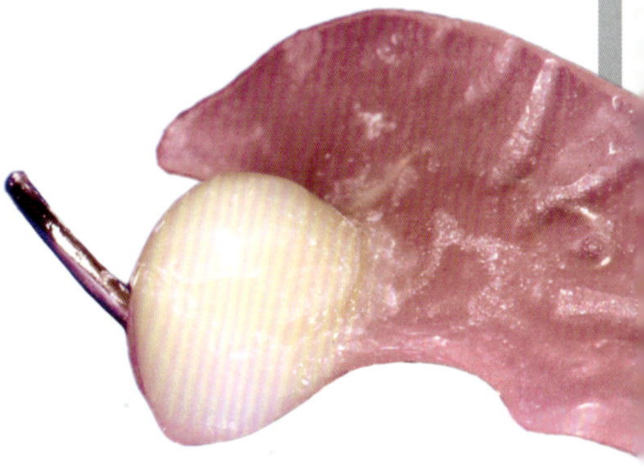

Fig. 30: Ovate pontic design of the tooth to be replaced in an interim denture

1.9.
Provisional restoration/ immediate restoration/ soft tissue contouring

1.9.1.
Provisional restoration after tooth extraction and during submerged implant healing

Even a provisional restoration after tooth extraction in the esthetic zone can make an important contribution to preserving the structure and positively condition the tissue in preparation for subsequent therapy.

Ideally, both fixed (Fig. **29**) and removable provisional restorations (Fig. **30**) should be designed with the replaced teeth as an oval bridge pontic ("ovate pontic") to provide optimal tissue support and prevent the gingival structures from collapsing. To do this, the bridge unit is sunk about 3 mm into the socket, depending on the height of the dentogingival complex. Procedures are also described in which the pontic is adapted to the socket in the further healing process and shortened accordingly [33].
If ridge-preserving measures were taken after an extraction, it must be ensured that the corresponding grafts are initially not subjected to any or only slight pressure by means of a correspondingly flatter basal design of the bridge units.

1.9.2.

Implant-supported provisionals / immediate restoration

Increasing esthetic demands as well as the effort to reduce treatment time have, among other factors, led to the integration of immediate restoration in the esthetic zone into the spectrum of therapy. Although such a restoration can be planned preoperatively, especially in the context of digital work flow, the restoration can ultimately only be reliably predicted peri- or postoperatively. In particular, the factors bone quality and primary stability represent the essential decision-making parameters [34]. With regard to preserving the marginal gingiva as well as the papillae, immediate restoration appears to be beneficial for single-tooth implants in the maxillary anterior tooth region [35].

Intraoperative analog impression taking (with modified drilling template or acrylic key)

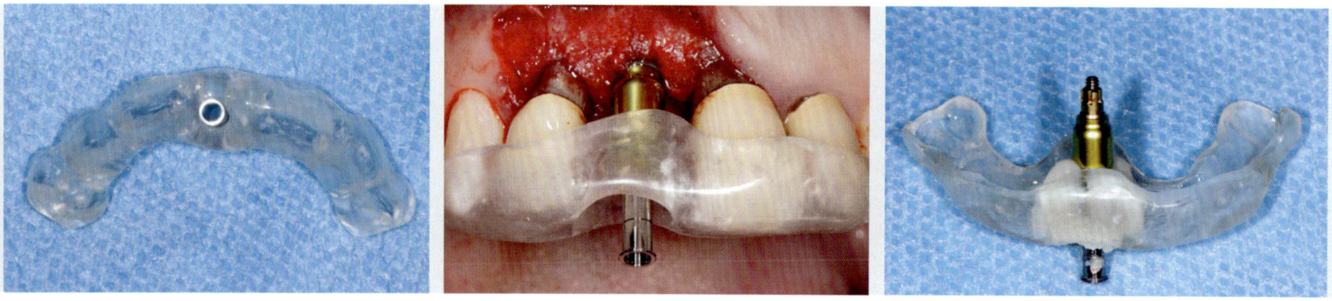

Figs. 31 a – c: Drilling template serves as key for intraoperative impression taking.

Digital intraoperative impression taking

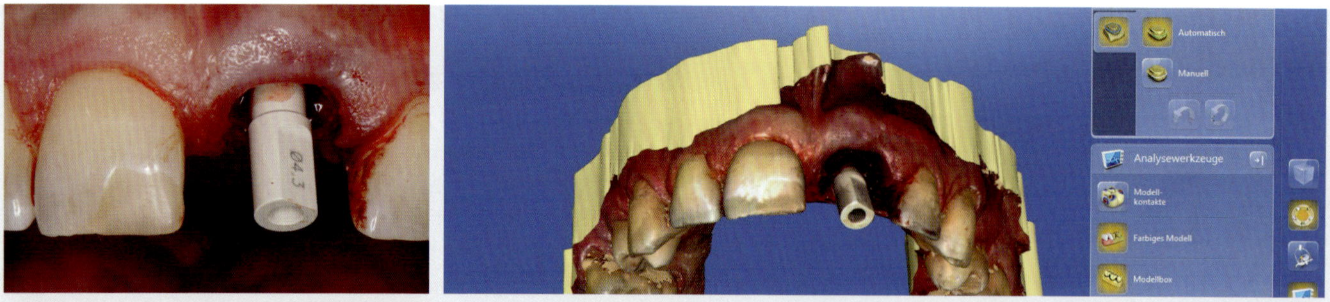

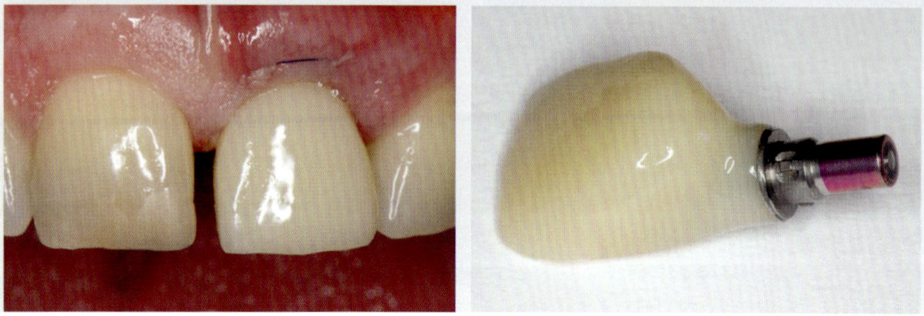

Figs. 32 a – d: Immediate implant placement, digital impression taking and restoration on the following day with a screw-retained temporary restoration on a titanium bonding base

Temporary metal or acrylic abutments, which can be further customized in the laboratory, lend themselves for immediate restoration. (Figs. **32a – d**).
The provisional restorations are screw-retained or cemented. In the case of cemented provisional restorations without prior digital surgical and prosthetic planning, composite copings prepared by the dental technician or a modified natural tooth crown can be adapted in a direct procedure chair-side on the corresponding temporary abutment. To avoid masticatory loading of an immediately restored single tooth implant as far as possible, prosthetic restoration should be performed in infra-occlusion and without approximal contacts [36]. Possible advantages of an indicated immediate restoration are a reduced treatment time, the usually already formed emergence profile, and possibly reduced treatment costs.
Likewise, after conventional, stress-free transgingival implant healing or after uncovering subgingivally healed implants, an additional therapeutic restoration in the form of an implant-supported temporary denture for shaping the soft tissue can significantly improve the predictability of the final result.

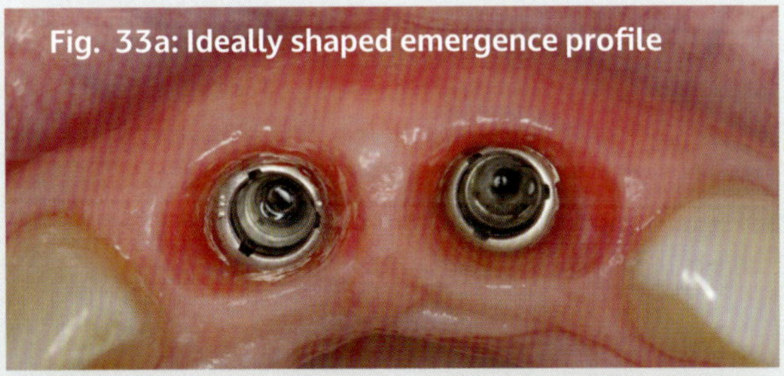

Fig. 33a: Ideally shaped emergence profile

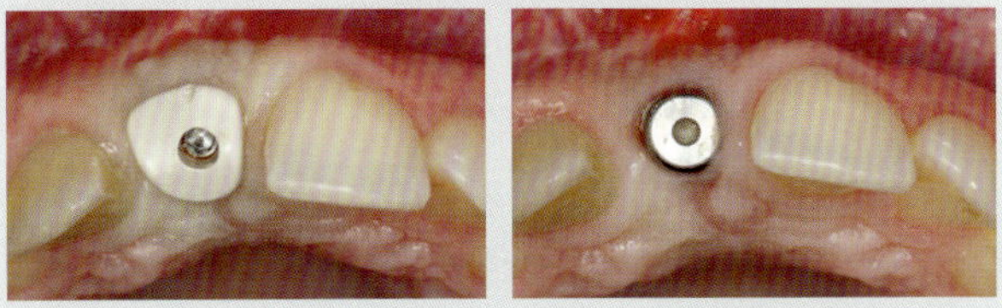

Fig. 33 b & c: shaped emergence profile with an individual healing abutment vs. a standard titanium healing abutment

1.10.

From a therapeutic provisional restoration to the definitive restoration

1.10.1.

Soft tissue contouring and transfer of the emergence profile using customized impression posts

Conditioning the peri-implant soft tissue directly after implant insertion or after implant healing and exposure using customized screw- or cement-retained provisional restorations or individual healing abutments can increase the gingival stability of the final restoration and lead to predictable esthetic results.
In general, an impression, a scan or a registration is required to fabricate the provisional restorations. Fabrication based on the digital three-dimensional implant planning data is also possible. Impression taking, a scan or registration is performed either immediately after implant insertion or after healing (transgingival healing) or exposure. This does not apply to immediate provisional restorations fabricated chairside. During the subsequent technical procedures, the dental technician can manipulate the gingiva on the master cast for an ideal emergence profile (Fig. **33 a – c**).
Whether the emergence profile is more convex, straight or concave depends on the geometry of the implant-abutment connection, the insertion depth, the insertion angle as well as the gingival thickness [37]. An emergence angle of more than 30° appears to be a risk factor for peri-implantitis [38].
In an alternative procedure, only a small amount of etching is performed on the model, and shaping is achieved by the clinician by successively applying plastic in several steps.
However, an attempt should be made to minimize these treatment steps while keeping the change of

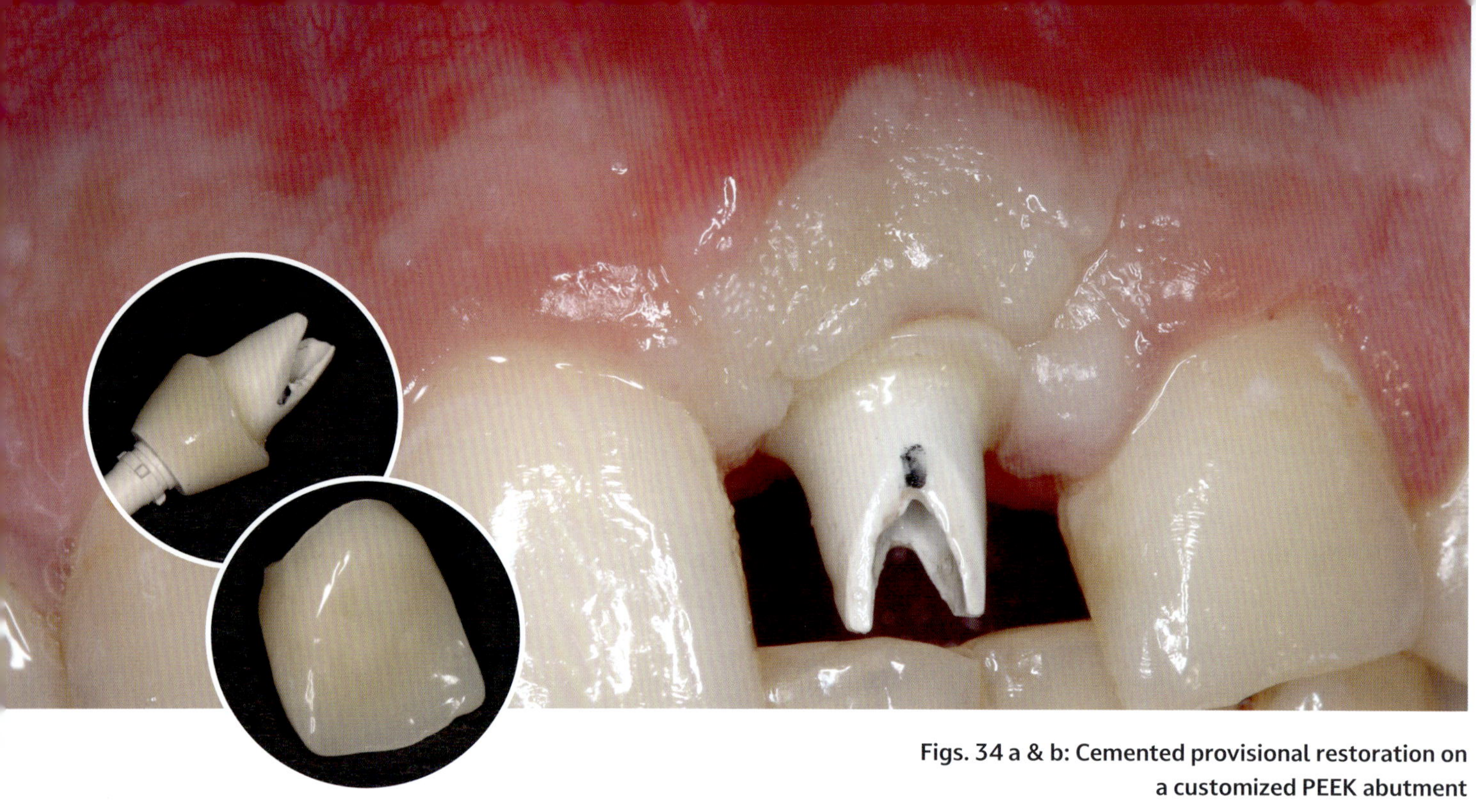

Figs. 34 a & b: Cemented provisional restoration on a customized PEEK abutment

Fig. 35: Forming of the emergence profile using a therapeutic restoration (note the change in color of the gingiva due to the pressure)

components to a minimum [39]. Likewise, care must be taken not to exert too much pressure on the vestibular gingiva (it should regain its color after about 10 minutes) to avoid recessions. (Figs. **34 a & b**).

After successful contouring, the desired soft-tissue funnel is obtained by removing the screw-retained or cemented provisional restorations. (Fig. **35**). The aim of the further treatment process is to transfer the designed emergence profile to the dental laboratory using customized impression posts that contain the information about the funnel geometry [40]. Due to the aforementioned problem of the soft tissue cuff around the conventional impression post collapsing, a precise transfer using conventional impressions is not possible

In conventional techniques, there are two different procedures for transferring the soft tissue geometry to the model:

1. The soft tissue funnel is filled with liquid plastic or impression material after unscrewing the healing abutment or the provisional restoration and screwing in the impression post. This must be done very quickly, as the soft tissue cuff collapses quickly.
2. A superior procedure is the fabrication of a customized impression post by "copying" the temporary crown. This post thus accurately transfers the emergence profile to the working model (Figs. **36 a – h**).

The transfer of the formed emergence profile is also possible within the context of digital work flow [41]. In the case study presented at the end of this chapter, this was achieved by means of a double-scan procedure [42] of the implant and temporary restoration, as well as subsequent data matching.

.

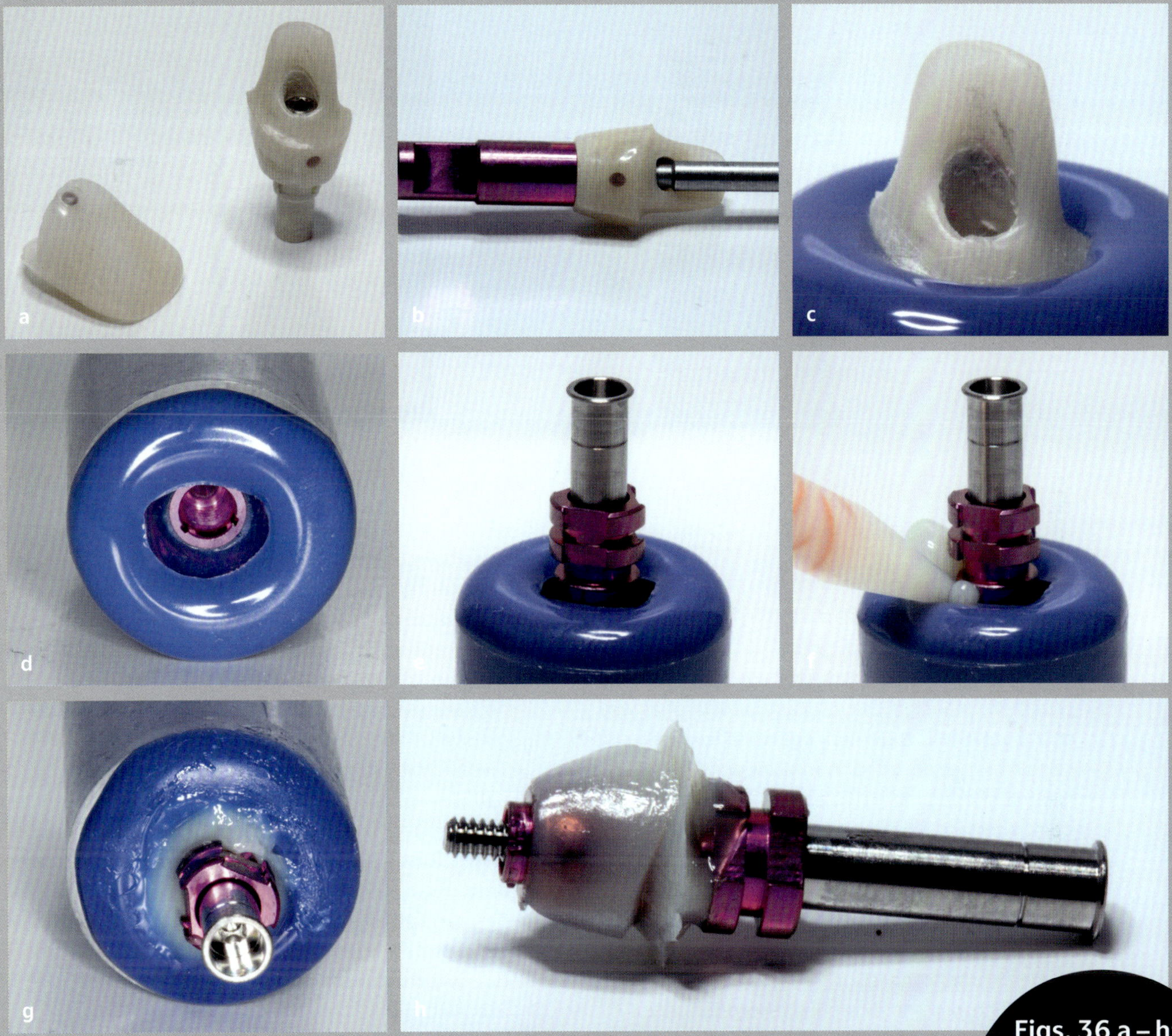

Figs. 36 a – h: Fabrication of a customized impression post

a) Customized provisional abutment with temporary crown
b) Abutment screw-retained on implant analog
c) Embedding in silicone for the purpose of taking an impression of the emergence profile
d) Shaped emergence profile
e) Screw-retained impression post
f) Filling the incongruent areas with resin
g) View after application of resin
h) Customized impression post prior to finishing

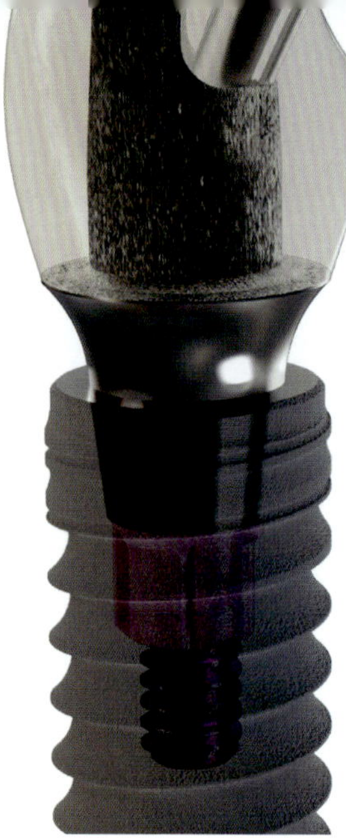

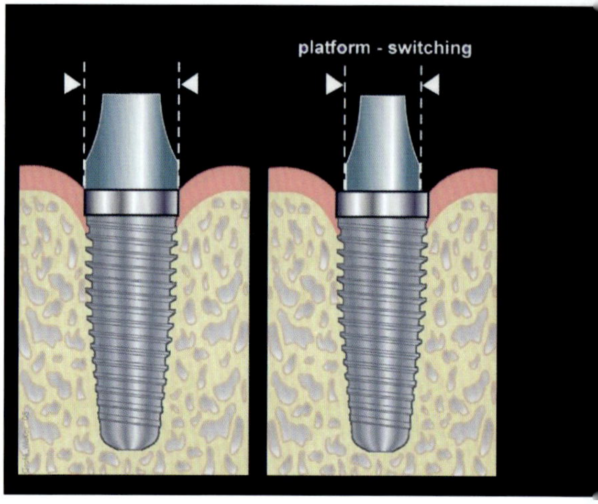

Figs. 37a & b:
"platform
switching"

1.10.2.
Definitive restoration

Beyond the surgical treatment steps that follow prosthetic planning, the "implant hardware" as well as the prosthetic treatment options allow for a certain degree of further optimization of the overall treatment outcome. In the area of the implant-abutment interface, "Platform Switching" (Figs. **37a & b**) appears to have a positive effect on the preservation of the crestal bone and stabilizes the peri-implant soft tissue [43, 44, 45]. A form-fitting implant-abutment connection, e.g. a conical connection or a "Tube-in-Tube" connection, reduces the pump effect in the microgap and thus bone resorption [46, 47]. The fabrication of customized CAD/CAM abutments made of zirconium oxide or lithium disilicate ceramic allows for the optimal design and implementation of the emergence profile in the final restoration and is currently regarded as the treatment of choice for single- tooth implants in the esthetic zone [48]. However, the manufacturer-specific abutment design plays a crucial role in terms of stability and long-term prognosis [49].

The abutments should always be tried in first before completing the crown in cemented restorations.
In this abutment try-in, the emergence profile and preparation margin are checked. To avoid subsequent recessions, care must be exercised to ensure that no excessive pressure is exerted on the vestibular gingiva.
The natural color effect on the gingiva [50] and sufficient functional stability in the anterior tooth region [51, 52] make zirconia abutments the first choice for single-tooth restorations in this indication area. (Figs. **39 & 40**). Abutments with a titanium base, so-called hybrid abutments (Fig. **38**), should be given preference over full zirconia abutments, as the risk of technical complications (abutment fractures, especially in the area of the anti-rotation lock) is considered lower for them [53].
A further advantage of ceramic abutments is the option of raising the cementing level without compromising on esthetics. Care should be exercised to use a fixing material that can be easily removed from the sulcus to avoid peri-implant inflammation caused by cement or adhesive residues, or to take measures to minimize this risk.

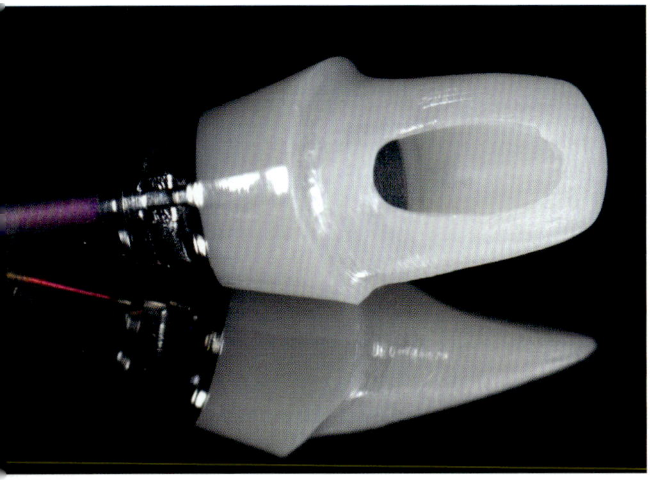

Fig. 38: Zirconia abutment with titanium bonding base

If possible and feasible, the directly screw-retained crown is a restoration option that is low in complications from a biological point of view, since bonding or cementing can be dispensed with. Even with implants that are angled more strongly towards vestibular, innovative therapy options enable screw-retention "around the corner" and thus a relocation of the screw access openings by up to approx. 22 degrees into areas that are not esthetically problematic. (Figs. **41 a – c)** [54].
In order to achieve functionally and esthetically perfect results in the esthetic zone, a close dialog between the dental technician and the dentist is essential, and the final result also depends to a large extent on the dental technician's skill. If pink-colored ceramic or stained and structured plastic is used to simulate missing hard and soft tissue as a makeshift solution, the success of this approach also depends to a large extent on the expertise of the dental technician.

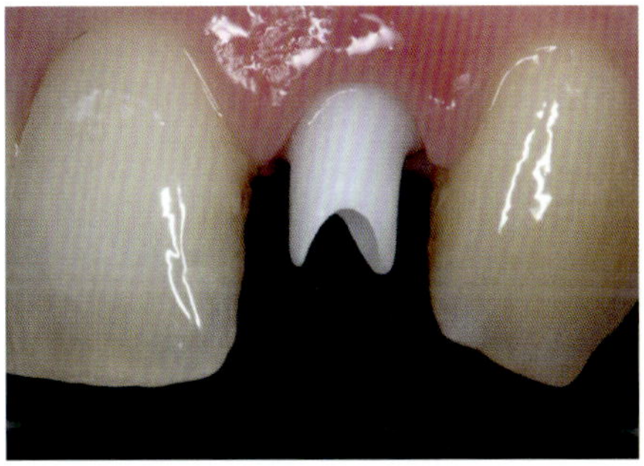

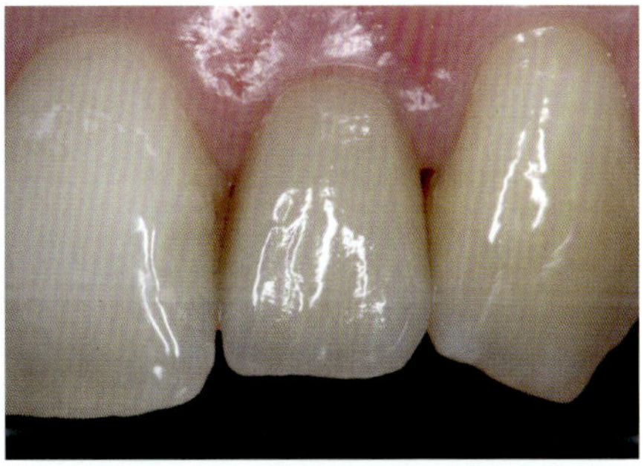

Fig. 39: Customized CAD/CAM zirconia abutment in situ

Fig. 40: Lithium disilicate crown in situ

Figs. 41 a – c: Angulated screw connection for metal-ceramic suprastructure 11

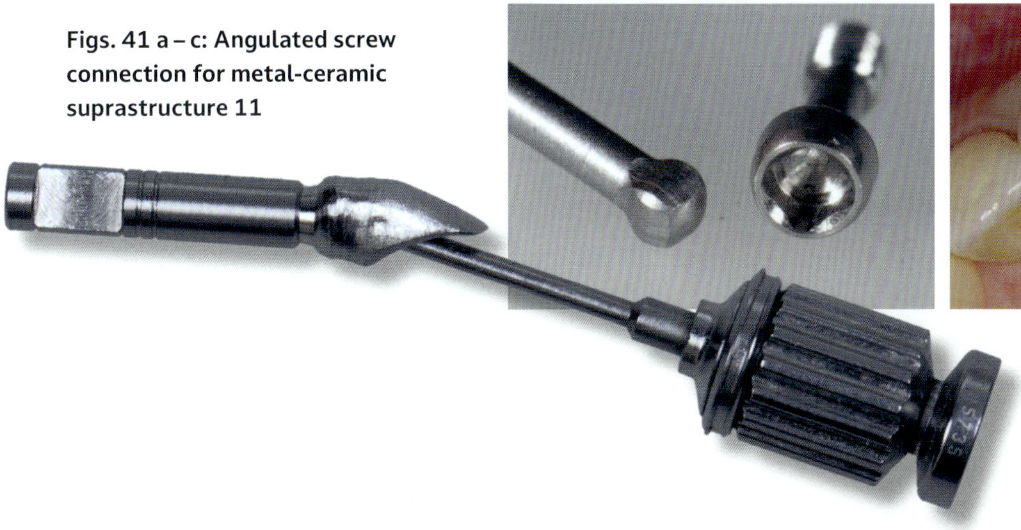

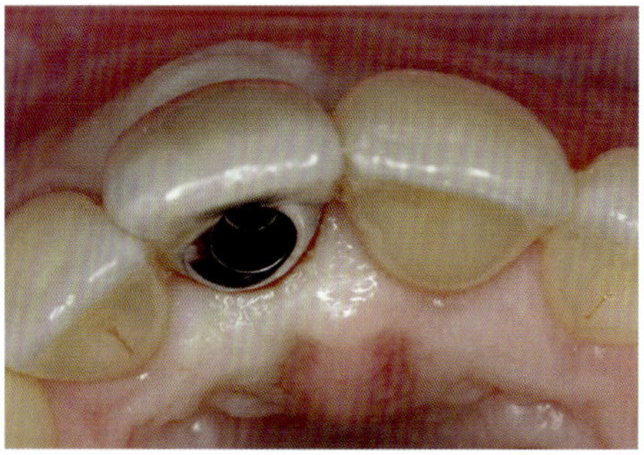

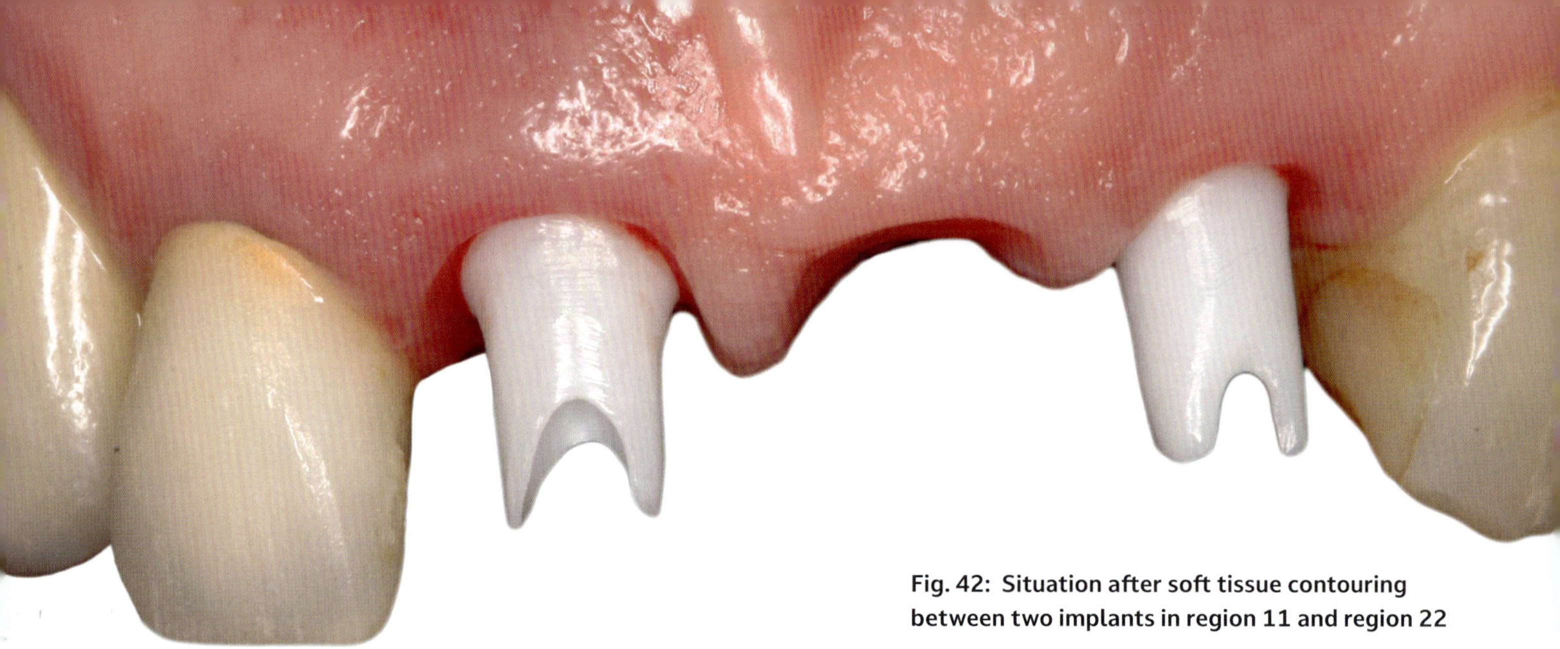

Fig. 42: Situation after soft tissue contouring between two implants in region 11 and region 22

1.11.

Multiple implants in the anterior maxilla

Replacing several teeth or two adjacent front teeth can be more challenging than replacing a single tooth. When multiple implants are placed in the anterior maxilla, the number of implants is also a factor in determining success or failure.

Tooth/tooth	5 mm/4.5 mm	Tarnow et al. (1992) Kois (2001)
Tooth/implant	4.5 mm	Salama et al. (1998, 2002)
Salama (2001)	3,4 mm	Tarnow et al. 2003
Implant/implant	3.4 mm	Tarnow et al. 2003
Implant/pontic	5.5 mm	Salama et al. 2004
Tooth/pontic	6.5 mm	Salama et al. 2004
Pontic/pontic	6 mm	Salama et al. 2004

Tab. 2: Possible average soft tissue height (papilla height) in various clinical situations (according to Zetu & Wang 2005)

In general, the studies listed in Table 2 confirm that two implants with a bridge restoration or cantilever bridge can be used to replace four missing anterior teeth more predictably than four individual crowns [55]. In particular, where there is limited transversal space, the insertion of four implants to replace four teeth can pose a problem. In terms of "red-white esthetics", the insertion of two implants, which may be combined with ridge-preserving or soft-tissue augmentative or soft-tissue conditioning measures in the pontic area (Fig. **42**), often provides better results. Even with two missing front teeth on one side, the insertion of only one implant in the area of the central incisor, provided with a crown and cantilever as well as possibly combined with ridge-preserving measures in the area of the lateral incisors, can prove advantageous. However, after extensive augmentation, several implants are occasionally indicated for functional loading of the augmented bone. A decision then depends on the clinical situation. A tooth-implant supported bridge can also be taken into consideration in exceptional cases if the abutment tooth/teeth in the maxillary anterior region are of good quality [56] and can be of advantage from an esthetic point of view.

Documented patient case "Immediate implant placement in region 11"

Fig. 43: Patient with a high smile line and tooth 11, that is not worth preserving

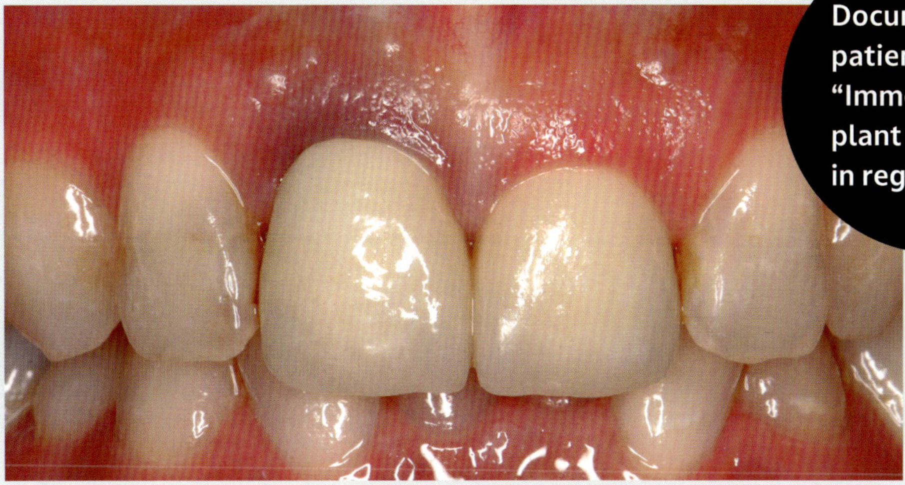

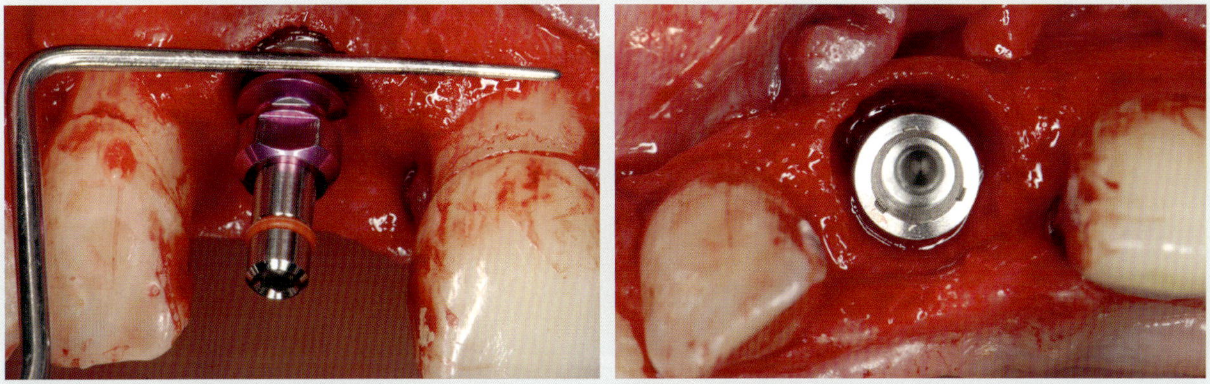

Figs. 44 a & b: Immediate implant placement while observing the correct three-dimensional implant position → aim for a palatal implant position!

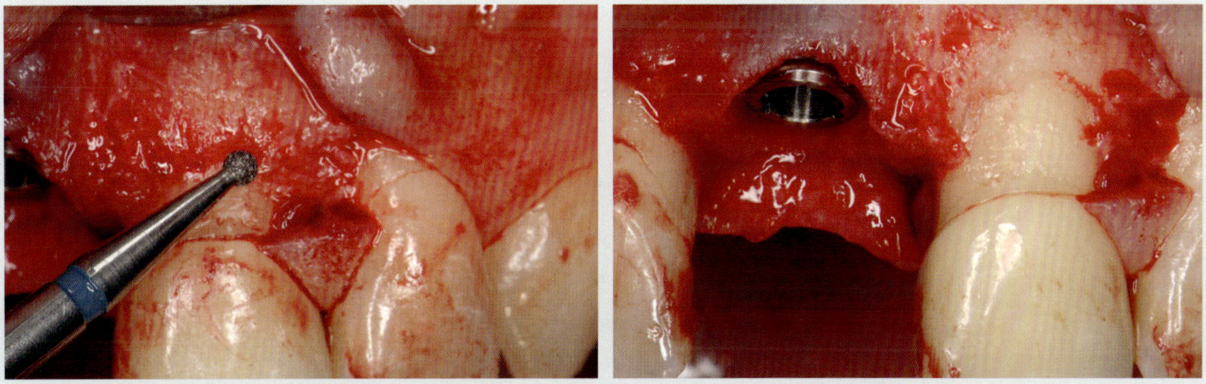

Figs. 45 a & b: Surgical crown lengthening on tooth 21 to create a harmonious gingival contour

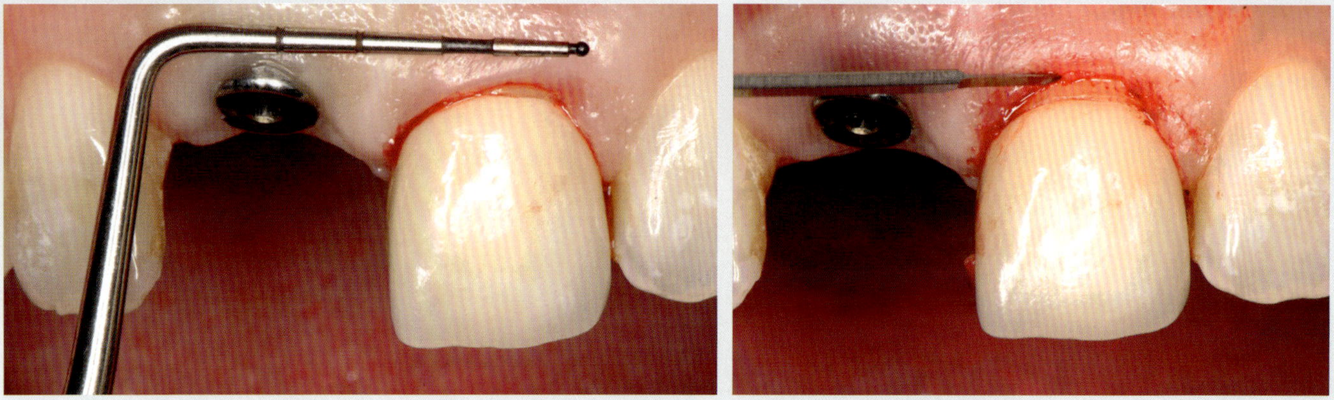

Figs. 46 a & b: Gingivectomy with a scalpel after a five-month healing period

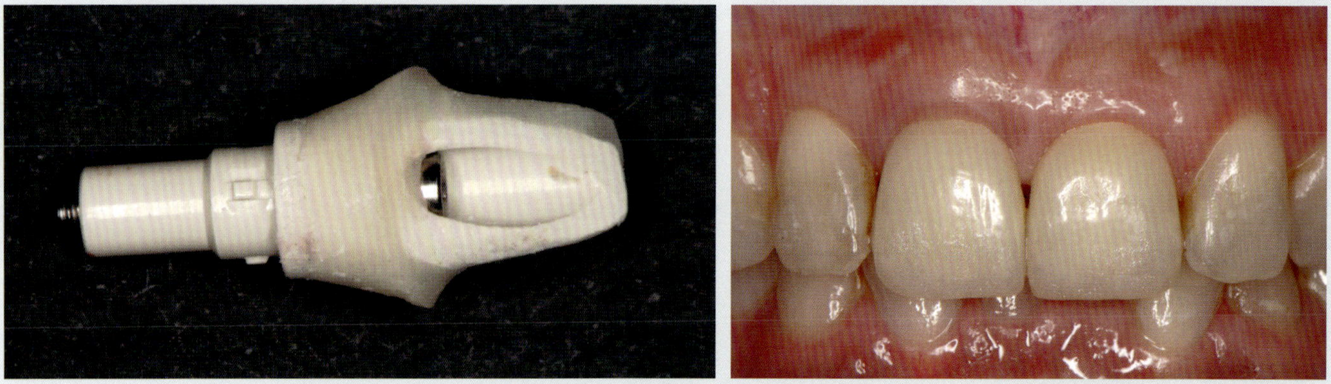

Figs. 47 a & b: Soft tissue formation using individualized provisional PEEK abutments and cemented provisional acrylic

Fig. 48: Formed emergence profile prior to impression taking using an intraoral scanner (not powder-free)

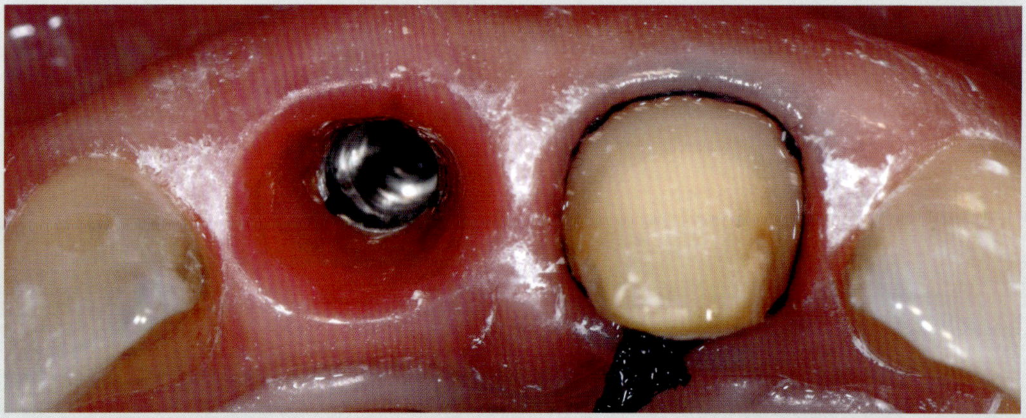

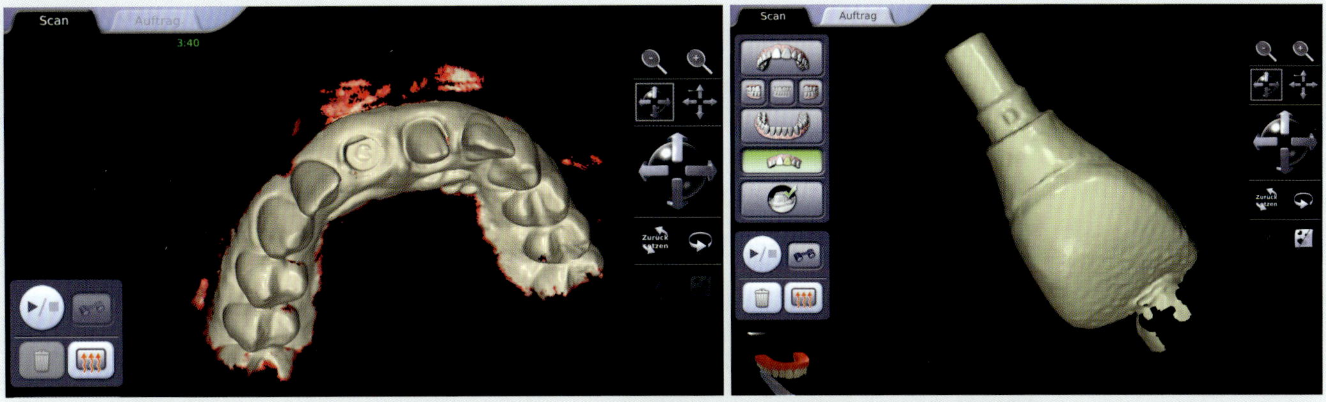

Figs. 49 a & b: Screenshots of the intraoral scan and screenshot of the extraoral scan. Using data matching of the two scans ("double scan technique"), the emergence profile could be transferred for fabrication of the abutment in a fully digital manner in the context of an individualized scanbody.

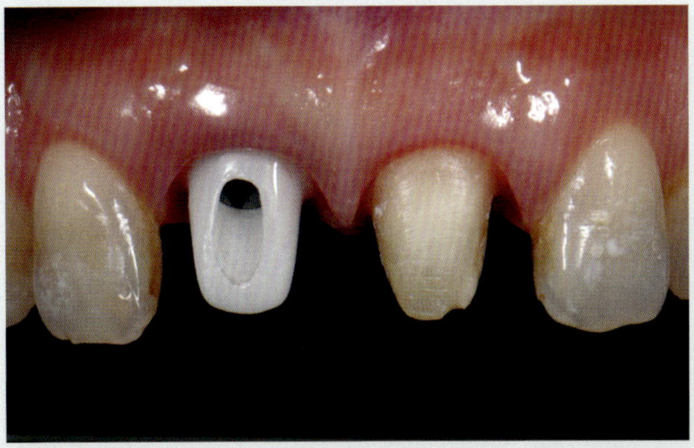

Fig. 50: Customized CAD/CAM zirconia abutment in situ

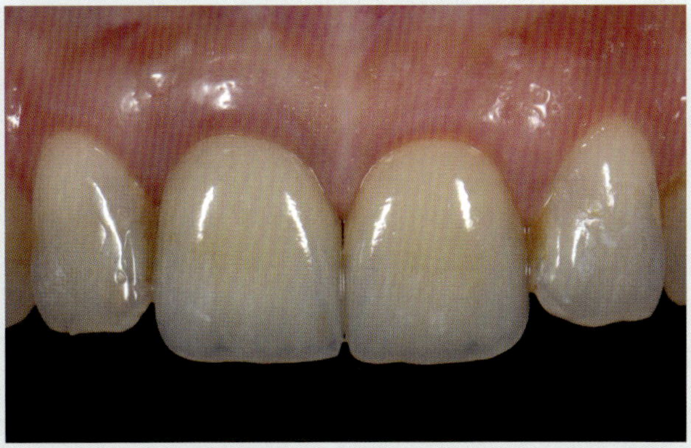

Fig. 51: Lithium disilicate crowns in situ

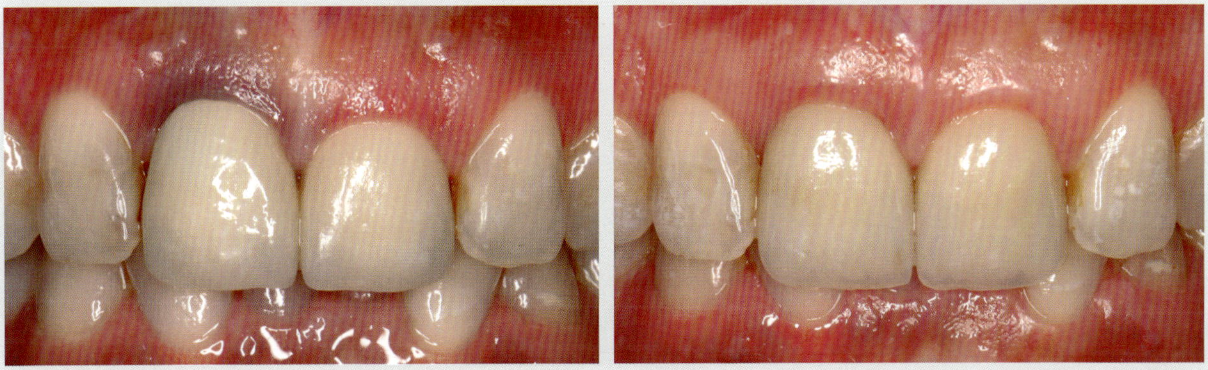

Figs. 52 a & b: Comparison of the preoperative and postoperative situations

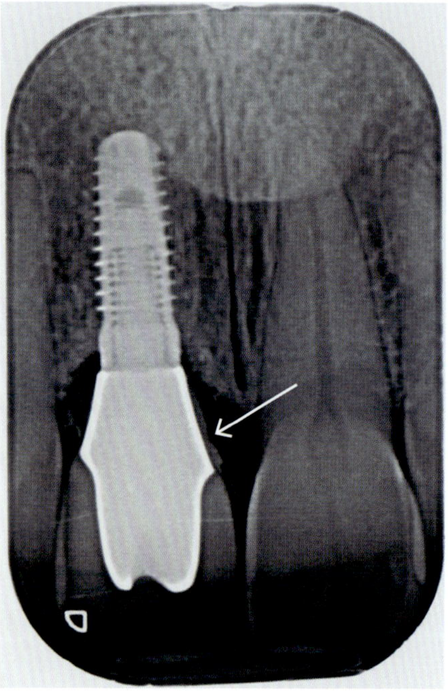

Fig. 53: Cement residue remaining subgingivally on the abutment after final cementing of crown 11

1.12.

Practical tips for managing complications

- In the case of remaining deep subgingival adhesive or cement residues, removal of the crown and the abutment and no curettage presenting a risk of deteriorating the soft tissue situation (Fig. **53**).

- In the case of recessions in the esthetic zone, if the implant is adequately positioned, there is no peri- implantitis and the recession is type 1 (see schematic overview Figs. **54 – 56**), then recession coverage can be performed under certain circumstances, preferably with autologous connective tissue [57 – 59]. The selected surgical technique must be adapted to the individual problem. Here, autologous connective tissue appears to be superior to the substitude material on the implant [60].

Schematic representation of recession classification on implants (without consideration of the orovestibular implant position) Figs. 54 – 56

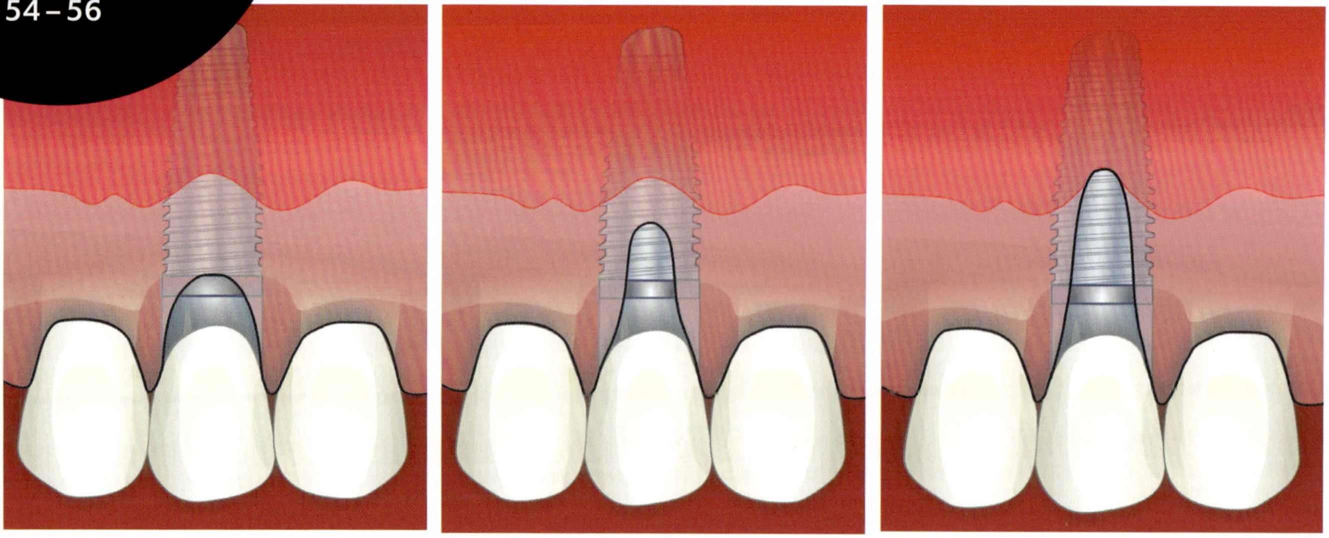

Figs. 54 a – c: Coverage possible (Miller classes 1 and 2/type 1 recession)

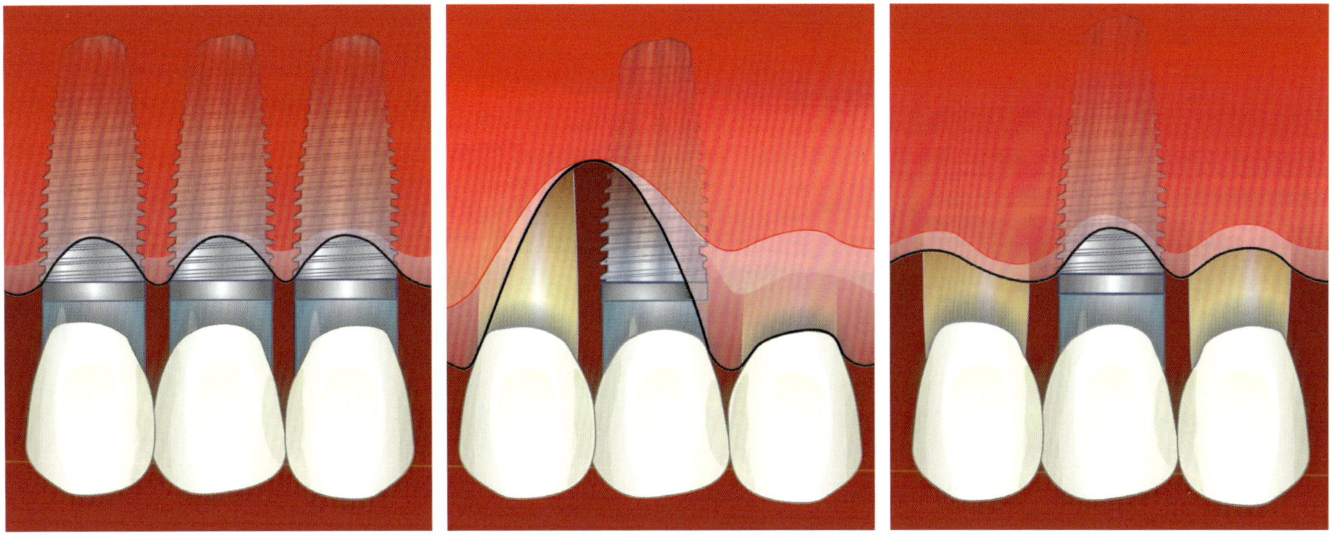

Figs. 55 a – c: Coverage not possible (Miller classes 3 and 4/type 2 and 3 recessions)

Fig. 56: Caution: peri-implantitis and/or recession?

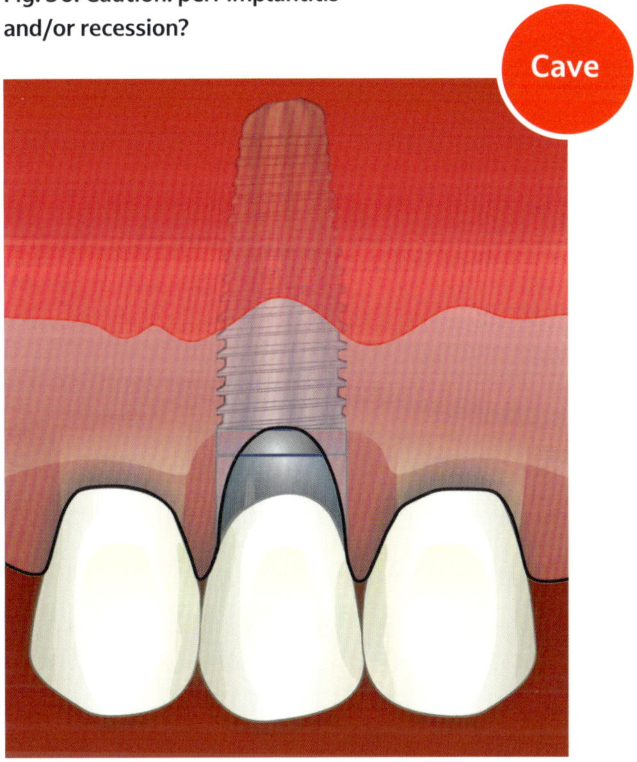

The limitations of reparative soft tissue augmentation are implant misalignments, peri-implantitis and type 2 and 3 recessions, which usually have their origin in previous peri-implantitis or periodontitis. It is particularly important to diagnose or rule out peri- implantitis, which is of course the priority for treatment. In cases of pronounced peri-implantitis or gross implant malpositioning, explantation must also be taken into consideration.

1.13.
Conclusion

For implant therapy in the esthetic zone, it is not advisable to dogmatically pursue only one therapeutic approach. The individual treatment strategy is based on patient-related factors, patient expectations and the requirements of the respective initial situation. The therapeutic approach should be as simple as possible for the patient, but as elaborate as necessary. Correct implant positioning and good peri-implant hard and soft tissue management are the keys to success. In challenging initial situations, and depending on the clinical experience of the dentist, it may be advisable to seek the assistance of a colleague with experience in this field of indication.

2

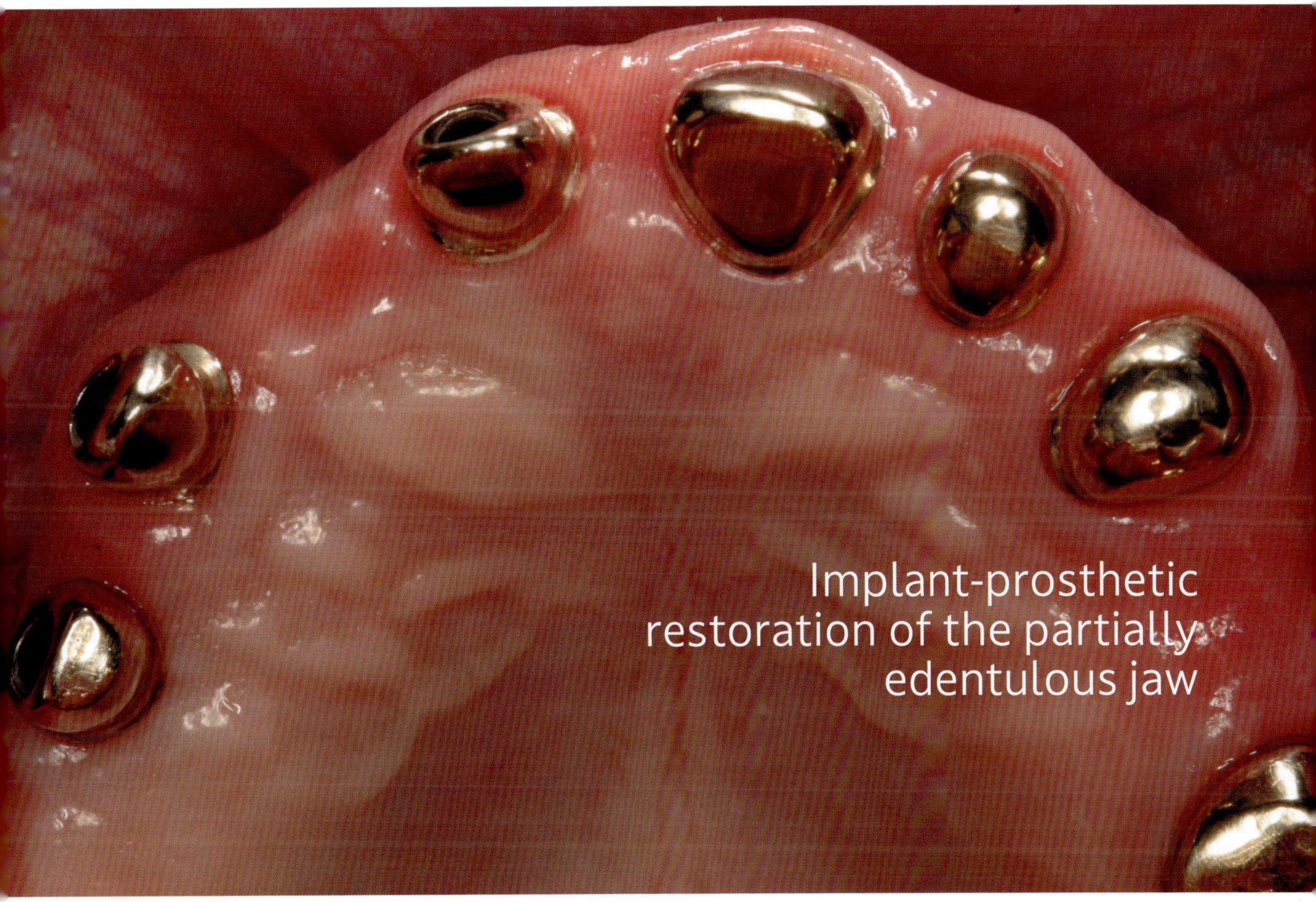

Implant-prosthetic restoration of the partially edentulous jaw

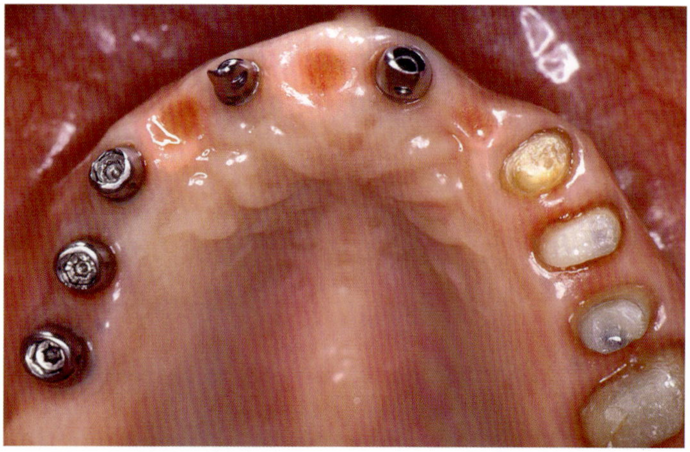

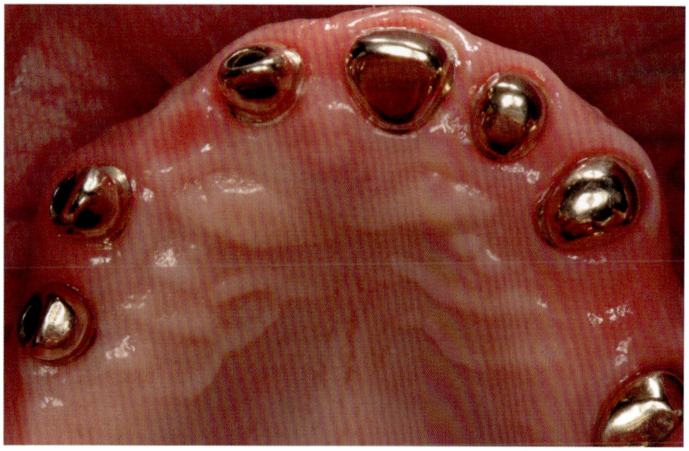

Figs. 57 a & b: Fixed or removable?

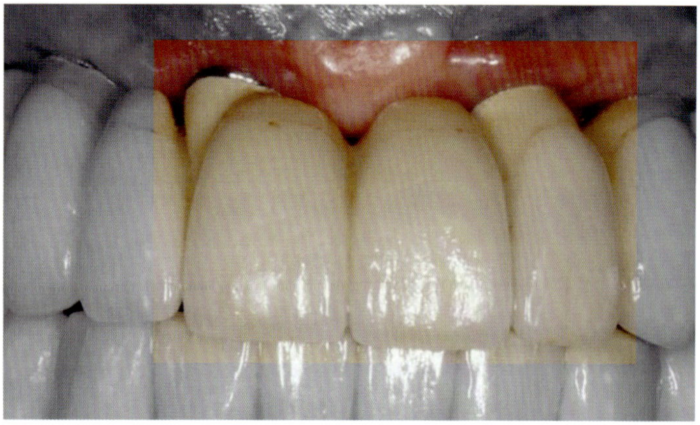

Fig. 58: Incorrect prosthetic implant position

2.1.

Introduction

Implant-supported restorations in partially edentulous jaws cover a very broad and heterogeneous spectrum. This ranges from single tooth gaps to free-end situations and severely reduced residual dentition with only a few natural remaining abutment teeth.

Particularly in the case of severely reduced residual dentition, the question often arises: "Fixed or removable?" (Figs. **57a & b**) In such a case, numerous factors influence the individual treatment method, for example, the age and state of health of the patient, previous treatment, the prognosis for the remaining abutment teeth, the extent of the loss of hard and soft tissue or previous periodontal damage, the number of implants, lip support as well as financial considerations, to mention just a few points. In partially edentulous jaws, it is essential that implant planning follows prosthetic planning in order to avoid malpositioning of the implants. (Fig. **58**). This requires thorough presurgical and preprosthetic diagnostics, and in complex and demanding treatment cases, consistent "backward planning" may also prove necessary. Of course, a fixed restoration is a goal that both patients and clinicians are keen to achieve. However, we can also see major advantages in removable restorations for older patients in particular, as they are easy to expand and clean. The following chapters are intended to provide an overview of the prosthetic treatment options in the partially edentulous jaw.

2.2.
Pre-implant diagnostics

The tools used for surgical and prosthetic planning, for example, include articulated master casts, intraoral scans, wax-ups, X-rays, DVT images, computer-aided implant planning as well as various types of surgical guides. (Figs. **59 & 60**). Minimal diagnostics involves an OPG image with a reference body, either an X-ray sphere or a prosthetic orientation template. In the partially edentulous jaw, implant insertion should always be performed with a surgical guide, or at least a prosthetic orientation template [61].

The digital workflows and planning software from various manufacturers enable consistent "backward planning" ranging from virtual implant planning to precision surgical guide with fully guided implant insertion through to immediate restoration. (see Figs. **61a – c**). However, certain deviations must be taken into account depending on the system, application and fixation [62]. It is not necessary to employ the same diagnostic effort in every treatment case, and even with the wide range of options available in the "digital workflow", a thorough "analog" inspection of the clinical situation or of situation models with regard to spatially conditions or the expected implant-crown ratio should not be forgotten.
However, three-dimensional X-ray diagnostics may be indispensable in the case of compromised bony conditions, unclear anatomical situations as well as for planned complex screw-retained suprastructures.

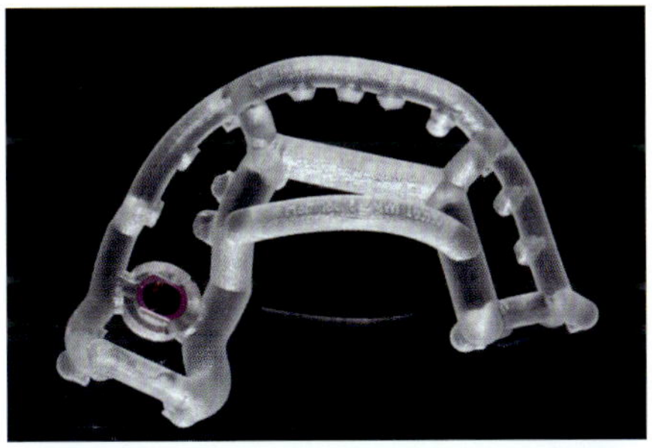

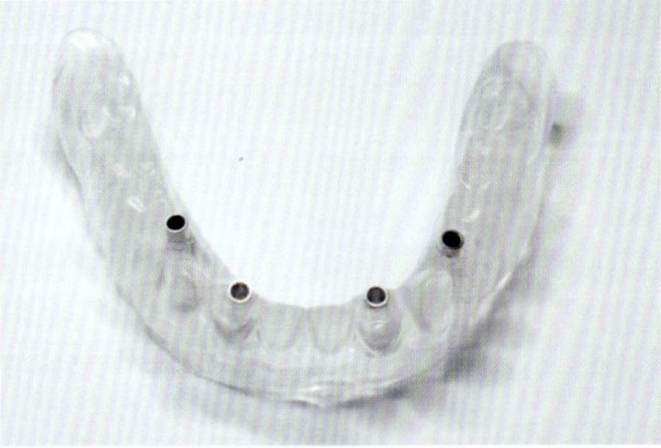

Fig. 59: DVT-based precision template

Fig. 60: Prosthetic orientation template

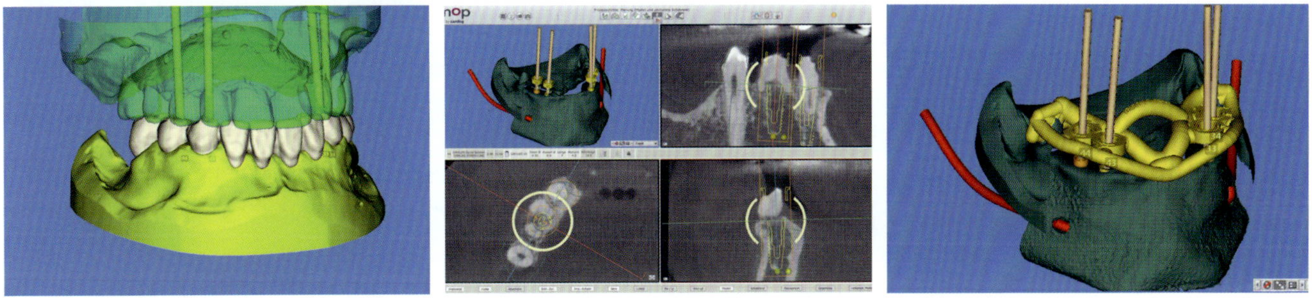

Figs. 61 a – c: "Backward Planning“ via digital implant planning and data matching.

2.3.

Fixed suprastructures

When it comes to implant-prosthetic restoration of the classic free-end situation (for example, from the first premolar) using fixed restorations, several questions may arise, which will be discussed in the following: how many implants are necessary [63]? Should the implant crowns be splinted [64]? Which material should we choose? Is the tooth-implant supported bridge an alternative? (Figs. **62a & b)**?
A low vertical bone volume or poor bone quality, e.g. following augmentation, may make it advisable to increase the number of implants. As a general rule, however, not every tooth needs to be replaced with an implant and, in the author's opinion, two implants are usually sufficient to replace teeth 44 to 46 [65].

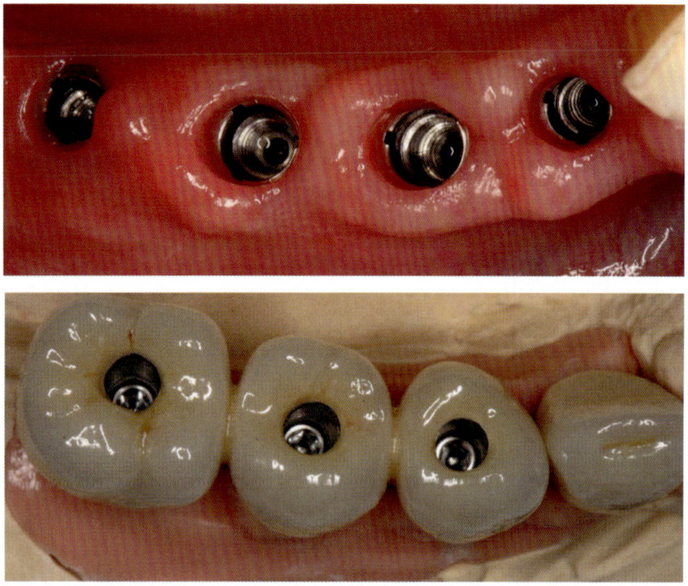

Figs. 62 a & b: Two, three or four implants? Splinting? Screw-retention or cementing?

Also of interest here is the observation by Fransson et al. that the center implant of three implants is most often affected by peri-implantitis [66]. In general, sufficient distance between the implants must be ensured..

2.3.1.

Splinting

An option in the case of multiple implants, is to design the suprastructure in the form of individual crowns or splinted crown units.
Various considerations play a role here: in principle, if the bone quality is reduced, the aim should be to splint individual units for the purpose of additional stabilization. A rather spongy or weak bone structure is particularly prevalent in the maxillary posterior region, especially following extensive augmentations or sinus floor elevations. In the author's opinion, primary splinting of the cemented or screw-retained crowns can in such situations prove beneficial.
A further criterion is the implant length, which can be limited by anatomical structures in both the posterior maxilla as well as in the mandible. This can occasionally lead to unfavorable crown-implant proportions, depending on the degree of atrophy, as the interocclusal distance has to be compensated for by the crown length [67]. From a biomechanical point of view, large crown heights are to be considered unfavorable, especially if the implants cannot be sufficiently anchored in the bone. In such cases, a crown splint should also be planned for reasons of stability.
The abutment-implant connection may also play a role here. Particularly in the masticatory region of the posterior teeth, which is subject to heavy loading, it is recommended in case of using an implantat system with an external connection to splint the crowns. Thus preventing prosthetic complications such as loosening or fracturing of the screws [68, 69].

A system with a stable inner connection ("Tube-in-Tube" or conical connection) is significantly safer to restore with single crowns and is less susceptible to translational forces.
Overall, care should be taken to ensure that several unfavorable factors do not occur at the same time in terms of bone quality, the number of implants and implant length.

What are the arguments in favor of splinting the crowns?

- Short implants and unfavorable crown-to- implant ratio
- Narrow implants
- Poor bone quality, augmentation
- Extendibility
- Bruxism
- Vulnerable external implant-abutment connection

Arguments against splinting:

- Absence of tension (the smaller the units, the better)
- Cleanability (can only be used as an argument to a limited extent when designing really good emergence profiles. Otherwise, interdental brushes must also be used for single crowns due to the larger proximal spaces)

2.3.2.

Screw-retained versus cemented

Crowns and bridges can be designed cemented or screw-retained (Figs. **63 – 64**). The clinical and technical procedures for cementing are similar to those for prosthetic crown and bridge restorations on natural abutment teeth, although for larger bridges, temporary cementing with Temp Bond or silicone- based, semi-permanent cements should be preferred. A planned screw-retained suprastructure generally places higher demands on the implant position than cementation, as the screw channel should ideally be located in the occlusal or palatal/ lingual area. (Figs. **65a & b**, page 44). If this was not possible, then mesostructures had to be used at least in the past, to which the crowns were provisionally or definitively cemented after screw retention.
More recent dental procedures offer the option of angulated screw retention, which allows the screw accesses to be placed in comfortable areas (see chapter 2.1.1. Angulated screw retention)
Of course, cementing and screw retention can also be combined in one restoration.

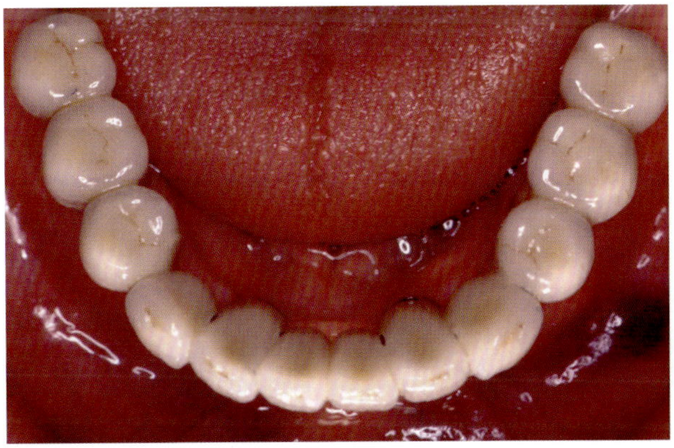

Fig. 63: Cemented suprastructur

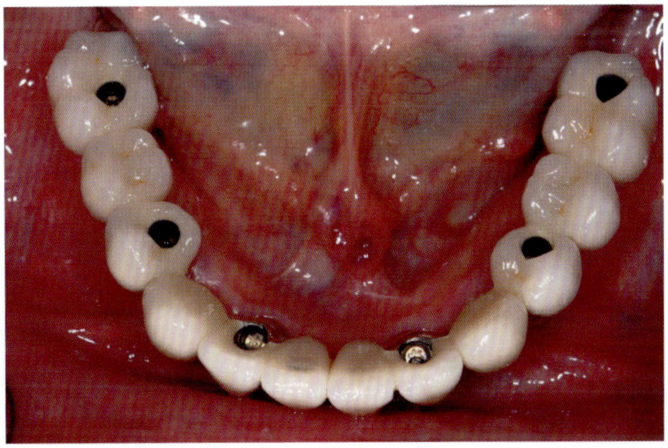

Fig. 64: Screw-retained suprastructure

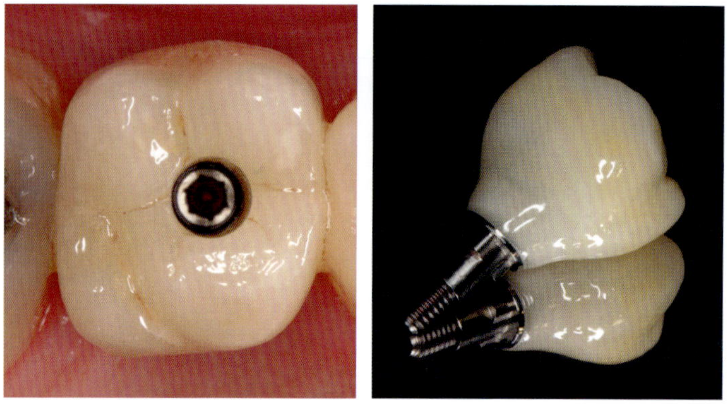

Figs. 65 a & b: Screw-retained lithium disilicate crown on a titanium bonding base

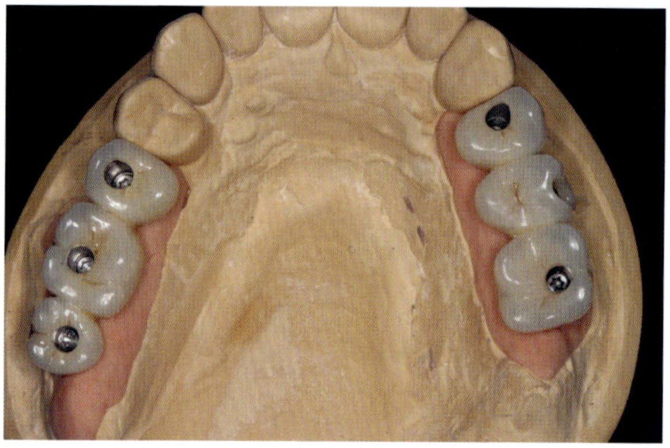

Fig. 66: Unfavorable position of the screw exit with a deviant implant axis in region 25

Advantages of the cemented suprastructure:

- Straightforward prosthetic planning and execution
- No compromised esthetics due to screw holes and less susceptibility of the ceramic veneer
- Sealing of any inaccuracies in fit with cement joints
- "Passive Fit“ [70]

Disadvantages of cemented suprastructures (in case of definitive cementation)

- Loosening of the abutment screw implies “trepanation” or destruction of the crown and possibly destruction of the internal thread and even implant loss [71]
- More difficult to expand and repair
- Risk of mucositis and peri-implantitis due to cement gaps that are difficult to control (cement residues) [72]
- As a rule, all-ceramic restorations must be permanently cemented.
- Visibility of the abutments in cases of recession
- Retention problems at small interocclusal distance

Advantages of screw-retained suprastructures

- Can be removed controlled at any time thus offering good repair and expansion options (Figs. **67a & b**)
- Time savings during insertion
- Fewer biological complications, as no cement residues can remain

Disadvantages of screw-retained suprastructures

- Occasionally problems with esthetics
- Limited in the case of suboptimal implant alignment and axis (Fig. 66)
- Weakening of the ceramic veneer of the occlusal surface due to screw access [73].

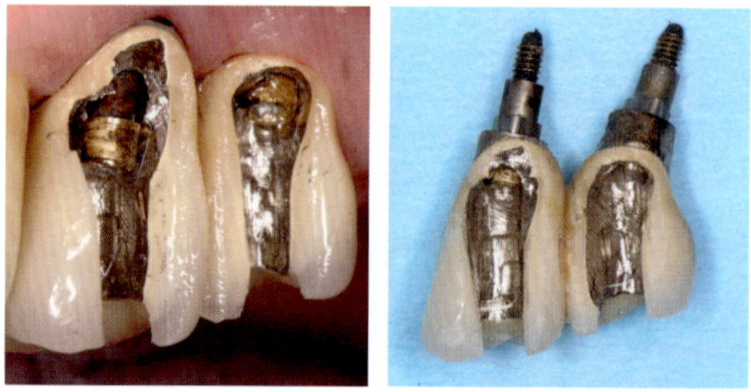

Figs. 67 a & b: Removal of two crowns after screw loosening

The realization of particularly complex large screw-retained suprastructures requires improved pre- implantological diagnostics and planning to be able to position screw accesses predictably in feasible areas. Complex backward planning, possibly using digital workflow, may then prove necessary. According to the review by Sailer et al. [74], screw-retained and cemented single crowns can be considered equivalent in terms of technical and biological complications.

However, for larger bridges, biological complications tend to occur more often with cemented reconstructions, so that a screw connection seems reasonable for complex fixed suprastructures. This also because the technical complications increase in this case [75] and, in particular, the risk of chipping increases with veneered zirconium bridges. If this tpye of restoration is choosen, the screw-retained connection should be clearly preferred [76].

In cemented restorations, the customized abutment is the restoration of choice, as the cement or adhesive joint can be moved to non-critical areas, thus reducing or minimizing the risk of cement-induced peri-implant problems.

With regard to the choice of material for fixed superstructures, the author continues to favor metal-ceramics, especially for fixed dental prosthesis. If, however, the decision is made in favor of all-ceramic bridges, they should tend to be of monolithic in design to reduce the chipping problem, which is thought to be even greater with implants due to their rigidity and lack of resilience (dissertation by K. Tokmakidis). Functional aspects as well as the condition of the opposing dentition should be included in these considerations. In addition to the treatment option of ceramic hybrid abutments or all-ceramic crowns on titanium bonding bases, whose long-term success is now well documented in the literature [77, 78], but certainly also depends on some specific dental technical factors, it is also possible to use customized abutments made of titanium or milled frameworks made of non-precious metal.

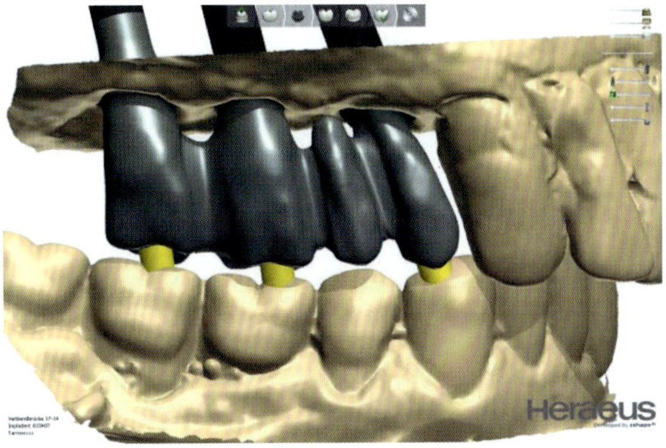

Fig. 68: Digital framework planning

In the posterior region in particular, the author believes that preference should be given to stability and functional load capacity. There, the metal-ceramic suprastructure can be superior in terms of stability, especially when technically vulnerable short titanium bonding bases are used in combination with ceramic abutments or crowns [79]. In the author's opinion, full zirconia abutments should not be used in the posterior region [80].

2.3.3.

Angulated screw retention

A desired screw retention places high demands on the implant positioning, as the screw accesses must be optimally located. Even with the aid of DVT-based surgical guides, this is not always possible due to the bony situation and would sometimes require extensive augmentation measures. In particular, labially inclined implant axes often result in the anterior and also in the atrophic edentulous maxilla, which do not allow the desired screw-retained restoration. New treatment options and digital manufacturing techniques (Fig. **68**) also enable direct screw retention on the implant shoulder in these clinical situations.

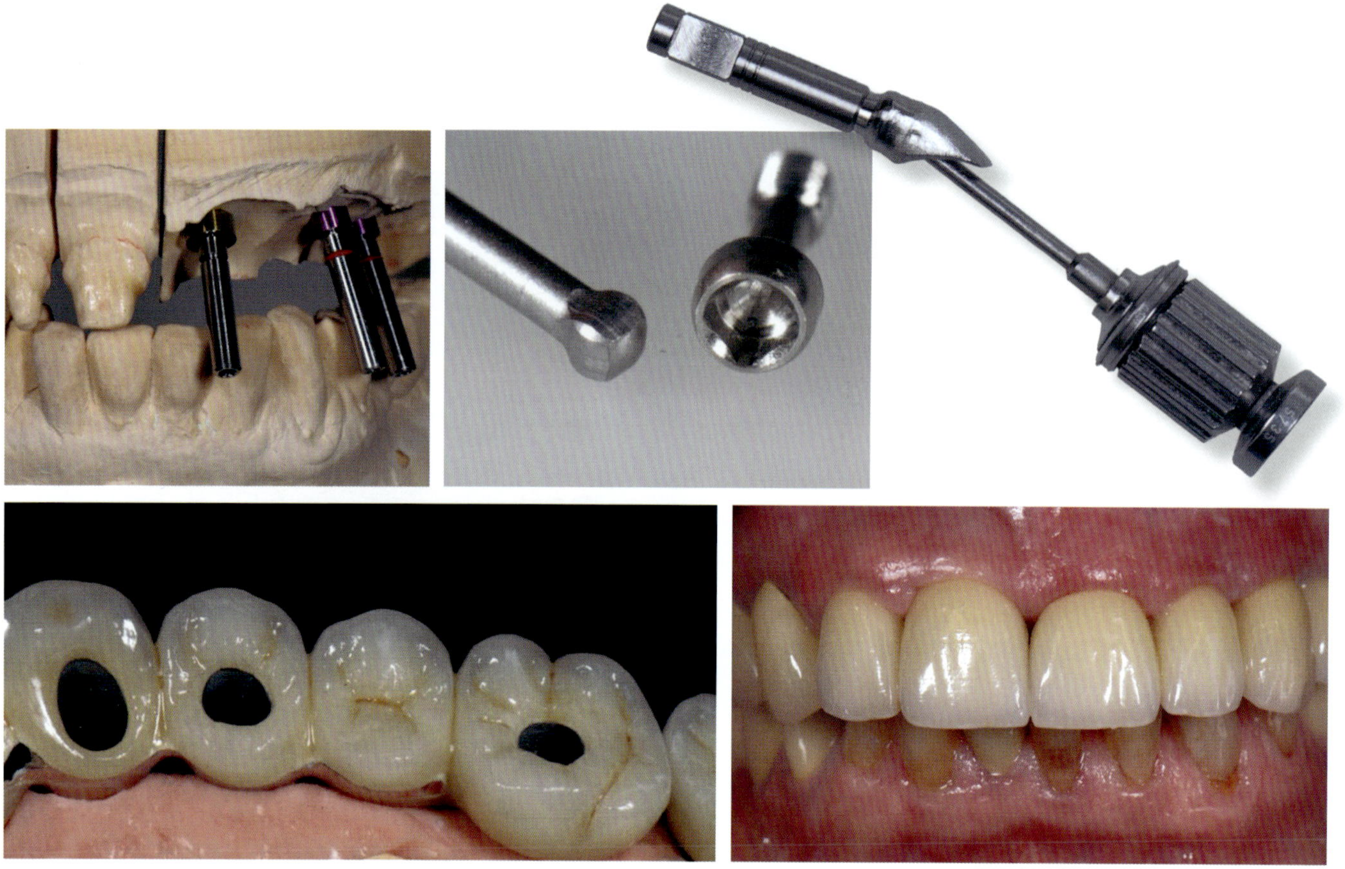

Figs. 69 a – e: Screw-retained bridge from 11 – 26 with angulated screw retention

By angulated screw channel technique using special screw systems, the screw accesses of the corresponding abutments or frameworks can be moved to the desired position, thus enabling direct screw retention where otherwise only cemented restorations or complex mesostructures would be feasible [81]. (Figs. **69 a – e**).
As these treatment options are offered by different manufacturers and companies and numerous special screwdrivers exist, it is essential to document the selected attachment for the benefit of patients and subsequent treatments.

2.3.4.
Tooth-implant supported bridge

Even though it is undisputed that the long-term outcome for a tooth-implant supported bridge is less favorable than for a restoration supported only by implants (80 versus 86% 10-year survival rate) [82, 83], it can still be a good and practical treatment option in many cases of free-end situations or the integration of natural abutment teeth into a fixed suprastructure [84, 85, 86, 87]. (Figs. 70 a & b).
In contrast to an implant, the tooth can be moved both horizontally and vertically.

At the time, this difference was the reason for the assumption that "stress breakers" should be used as compensation elements in reconstructions con-

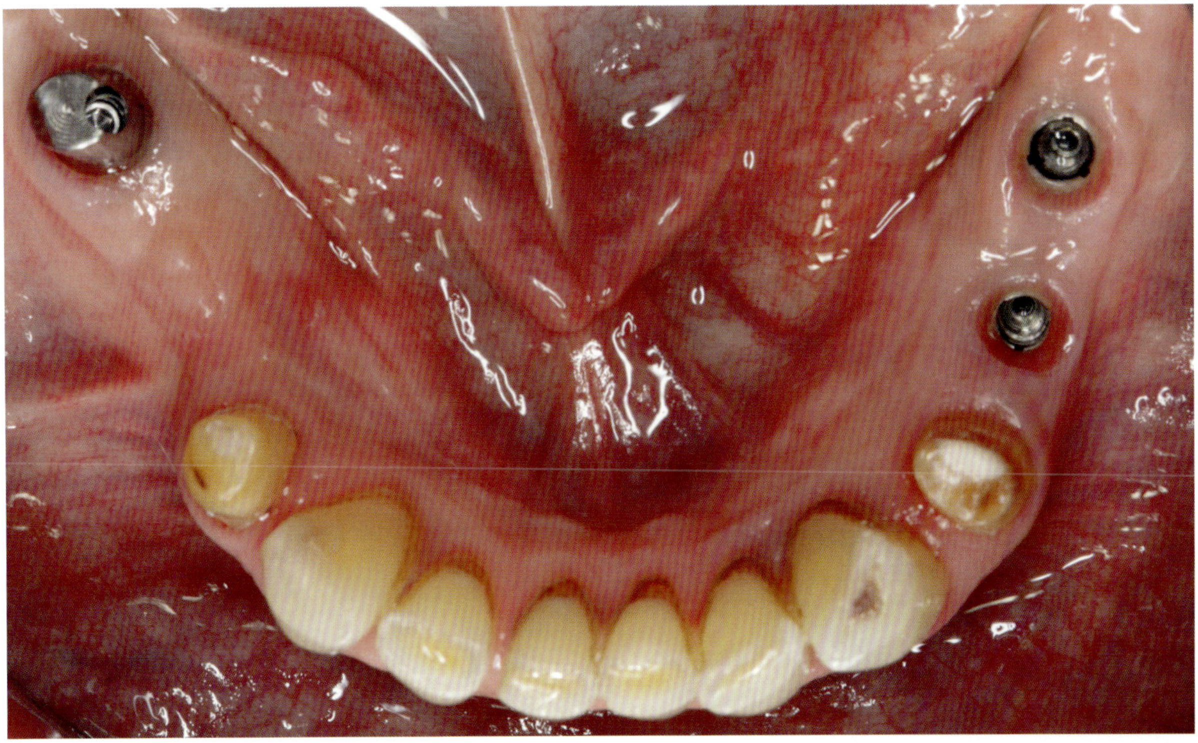

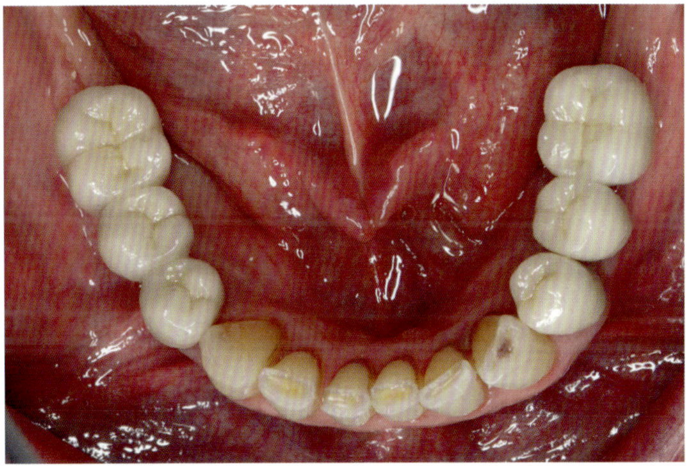

necting tooth and implant, such as the intramobile elements made of plastic in the former IMZ implant. Richter et al. examined the connection between teeth and implants in vivo from a biomechanical point of view [88]. In this process, masticatory force measurements were taken using force measuring cells in the implant abutment parts of IMZ implants. It was demonstrated that hardly any notable intrusive movement occurs due to the impulsive application of force under normal masticatory loading of a tooth. At low loads, the difference in rigidity between the abutment tooth and the implant has no effect (e.g. dental arch occlusion). In the case of short-term high, functionally-caused vertical loads, the resilience of teeth and implants becomes aligned because blood and intercellular fluid cannot flow out of the periodontal tissue.

Figs. 70 a & b: Tooth-implant supported bridge and purely implant-supported crowns

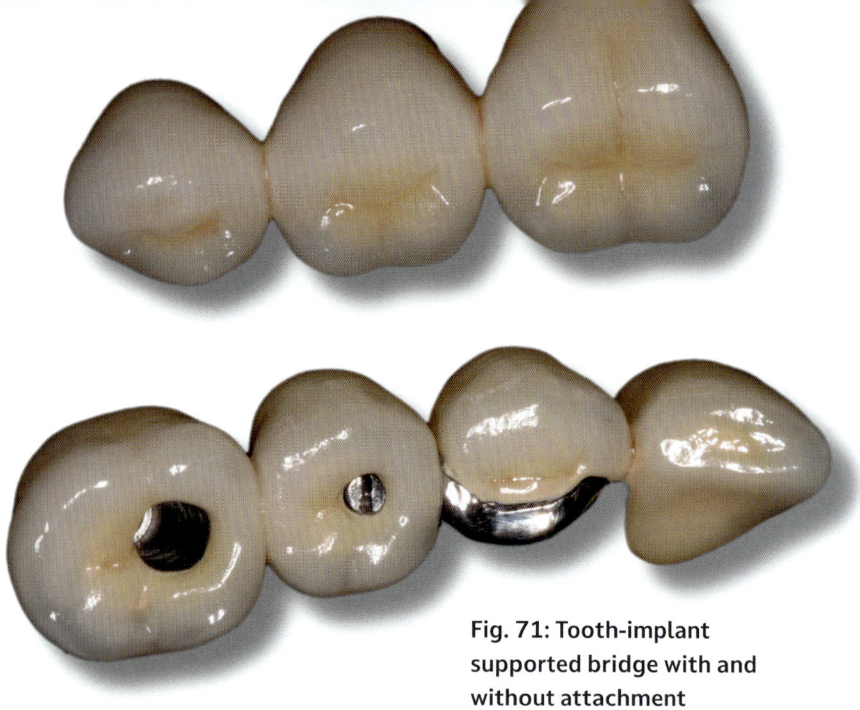

Fig. 71: Tooth-implant supported bridge with and without attachment

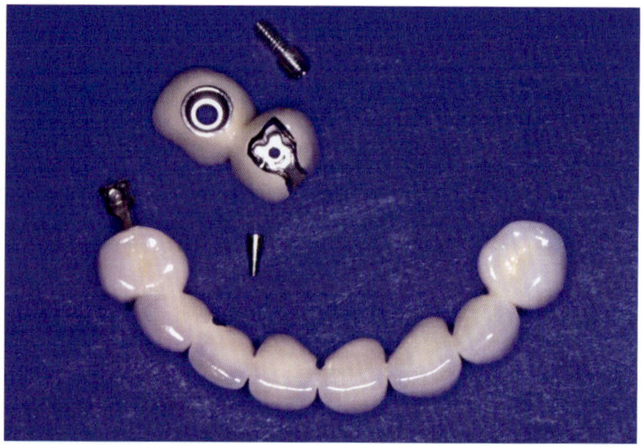

Fig. 72: Segmented tooth-implant supported bridge with attachment

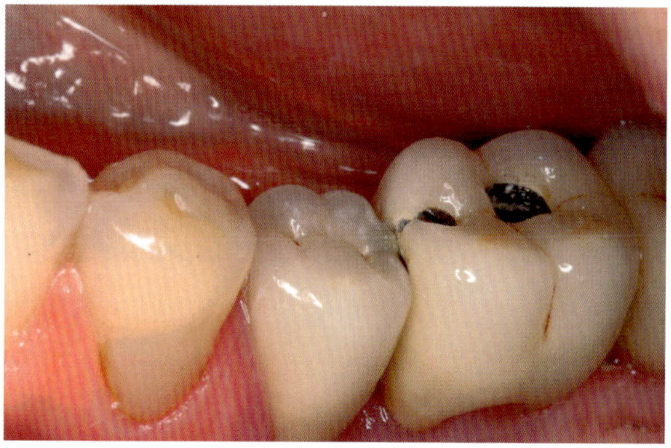

Fig. 73: Tooth intrusion after fracture of a previously rigid attachment

The intrusion of the tooth did not result in a bending load on the implant. From a biomechanical point of view, teeth and implants can therefore be considered equivalent in terms of their functional load-bearing capacity [89].
However, particular attention should be paid to the quality of the natural abutment tooth or teeth: the abutment tooth in a tooth-implant supported bridge should be clinically stable. Furthermore, it is advantageous if the terminal tooth has not been treated endodontically. Teeth with post and core build- ups as the sole abutment, especially in the absence of a "ferrule effect" (barrel hoop effect in the preparation of post build-ups), should be avoided.

Tooth-implant supported bridges are suitable treatment options for free-end situations or shortend dental arch if:

- due to unfavorable anatomical conditions, only one implant can be anchored and extensive augmentation is to be avoided,
- due to financial considerations, for example, reduced planning is necessary,
- there is a need for treatment of the end tooth (crown).

In principle, there are several options for a restoration:

- **Segmented tooth-implant supported bridge**
  In this case, a screw-retained connection is made in the implant combined with a rigid, screw-retained extra-coronal attachment on the terminal tooth, possibly with circumferential milling on the lingual/palatal section of the definitively cemented anchor crown.(Figs. **71 – 72**). This type of restoration is rarely chosen these days, but it can certainly have advantages - especially when periodontal interventions on the implant are necessary.

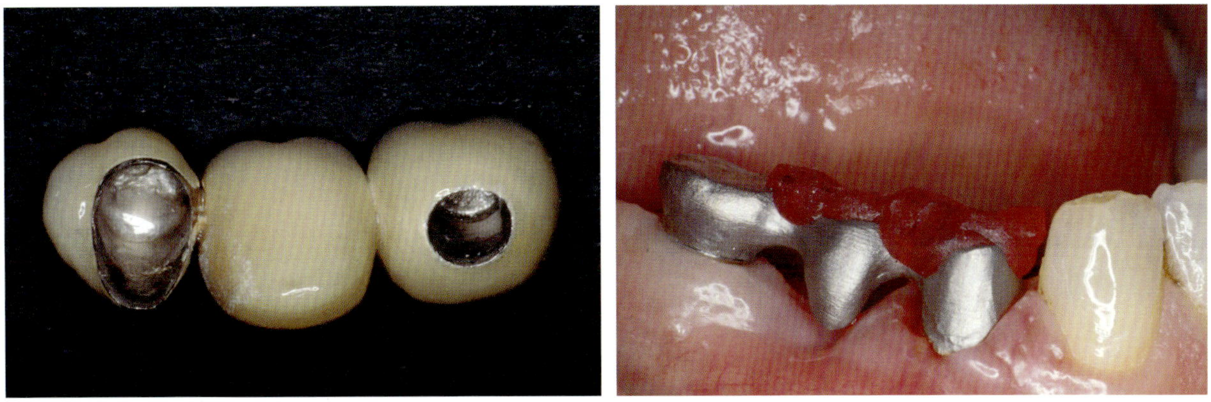

Figs. 74 a & b: Conventionally cemented tooth-implant supported bridge

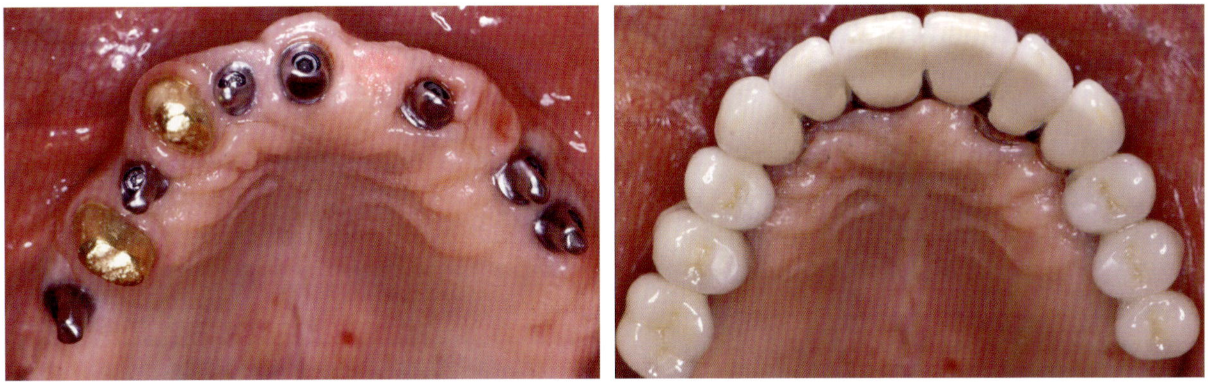

Figs. 75 a & b: "Greifswald tooth-implant supported bridge" with galvano caps at 13 and 15

In principle, it should be noted that a rigid tooth-implant supported bridge is chosen, as the use of non-rigid connecting elements (e.g. non-screw- retained attachments) entails a risk of intrusion of the natural abutment tooth. (Fig. **73**). When the tooth is subjected to pressure, the parts of the attachment may become jammed, causing the tooth to “submerge”; which cannot be reset during the pressure-free interval.

- **Conventionally cemented or cemented/ screw-retained bridge designs**
  The bridge is either cemented to the tooth and abutment or cemented to the tooth and screw-retained to the implant. (Figs. **74 a & b**).

- **"Greifswald tooth-implant supported bridge"** [90]
  The design is created such that the natural abutment tooth is restored with a definitively cemented galvano cap and then the bridge is provisionally cemented onto the implant and galvanic framework (Figs. **75 a & b**) or cemented to the tooth and screw-retained on the implant.
  With the help of the galvano or thin metal caps, natural abutment teeth can be easily integrated into provisionally cemented or screw-retained restorations, thus being protected against caries.

2.4.

Removable suprastructures/ strategic increase in the number of abutments

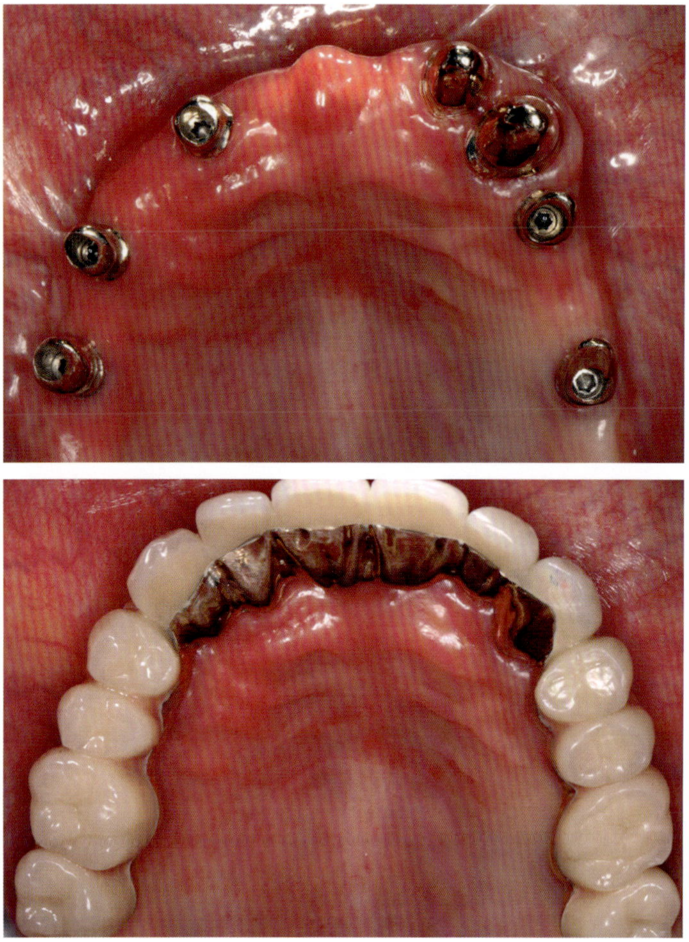

Figs. 76 a – b: Tooth/implant-supported telescopic bridge

The telescope technique is particularly recommended for removable restorations in partially edentulous jaws. This way, natural teeth and implants can be combined in one restorative framework.

The concept of a strategic abutment increase is a prosthetic-implant-based treatment concept for severely reduced residual dentition. Implants offer the possibility of supporting or stabilizing a reduced number of remaining teeth worthy of preservation in strategic positions in the context of increasing abutments. The implants are inserted into key prosthetic and biomechanical positions within the dental arch. (Figs. **76 a & b**). This approach ensures that removable partial dentures and telescopic bridges are optimally supported, and in fact makes such restorations possible in the first place. The statics of the denture, comfort and resilience of the suprastructure can thus be improved [91]. The implants should not be undersized in this area. The teeth involved should be firm and have a good long- term prognosis both periodontally and prosthetically.
The treatment concept can also be considered beneficial in terms of the longevity of the restoration [92, 93, 94]. Ideally, a quadrangular, but at least a rectangular, linear support running perpendicular to the alveolar ridge is aimed for. (Figs. **77 a – e** and **81 a & b**). Depending on the number of abutments, the telescopic crowns are used to support removable partial dentures (tooth-/implant-supported and mucosa-supported suprastructures, see Figs. **81 a & b**), possibly with lingual or palatal connectors or telescopic bridges without palate cover and sublingual bracket. (Figs. **76 a & b**).

Examples of support in the context of increasing the number of abutments (Figs. 77a – e)

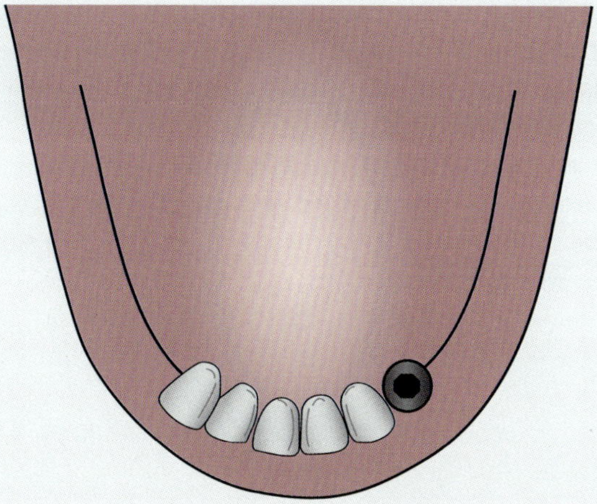

a

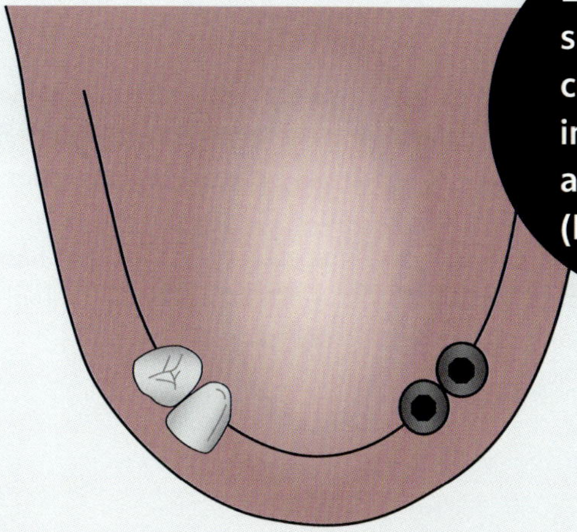

b

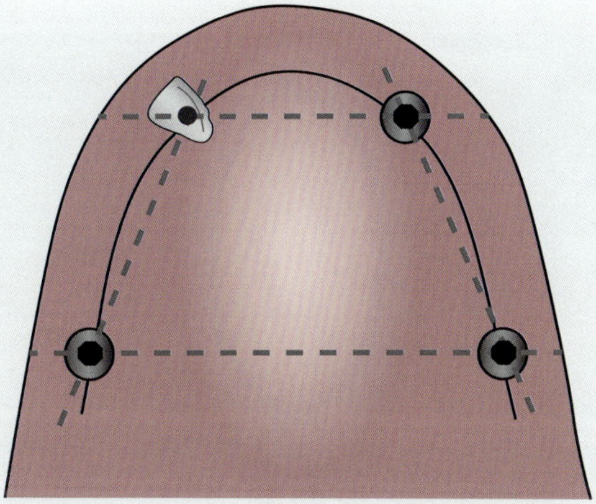

c

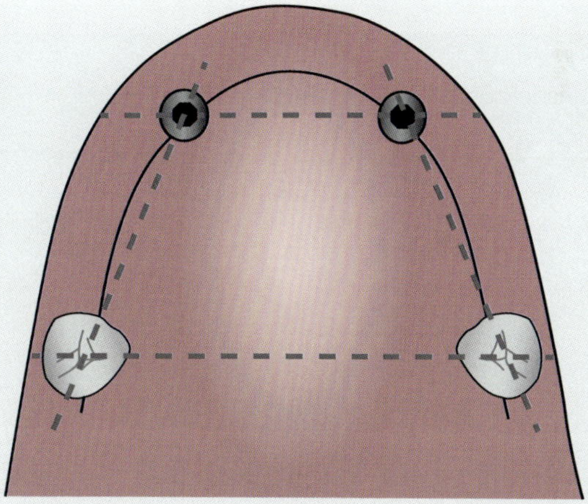

d

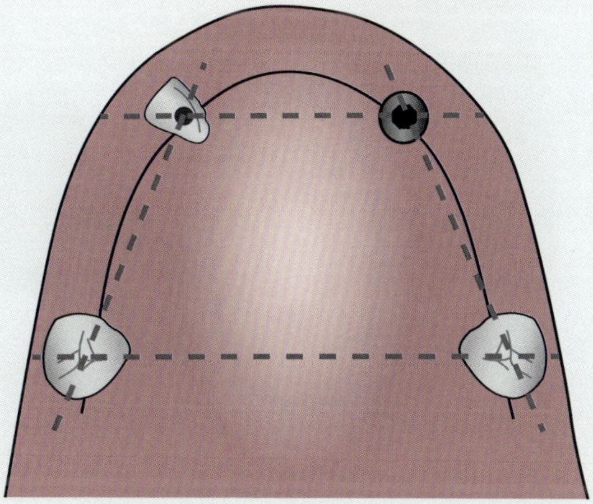

e

Figs. 77 a – e: Options of prosthetic support in the context of increasing abutment numbers

Advantages of the treatment concept:

Telescopic bridges and partial dentures have many advantages, especially in the long term: if a tooth or implant is lost at a later date, the entire restoration can be expanded easily, and this process could repeated several times if necessary. On the other hand, it is also possible to incorporate additional implant abutments into existing dentures.

This treatment concept is therefore characterized by particular cost-effectiveness. Another advantage is the good hygienic capability, especially for older patients. The surgical treatment effort is usually manageable, and extensive augmentations can be avoided, as transversal or vertical tissue deficits can be compensated for by means of labial resin shields as well as saddles.

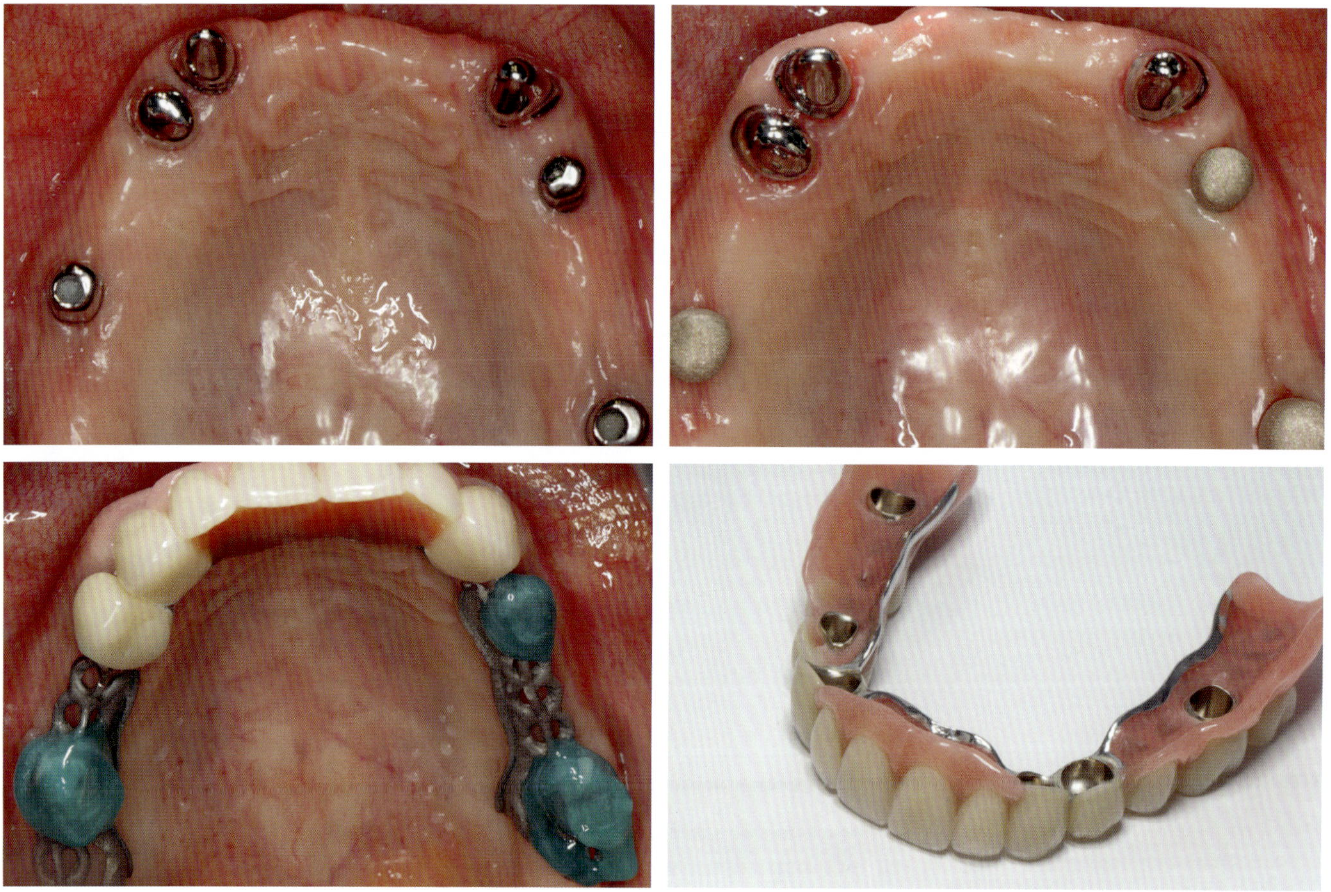

Figs. 78 a – d: Intraoral bonding of the casted thin crown-caps, placed on the implant abutments, with the metal-cast for a "Passive Fit“

The necessity of a labial shield for soft tissue support can also make a removable bridge unavoidable from an esthetic point of view, even if there is a sufficient number of abutments for a fixed restoration.
In selected situations, the inserted abutments can also be fitted with locators or ball abutments. This makes an expansion even more cost-effective and easier.

However, retention and guidance are not necessarily comparable to a full-fledged telescope.
Furthermore, it should be noted that the different removal path of a telescope and locator (bending) leads to increased stress on the contralateral tooth/teeth. In situations as shown in the Figures **79 a & b** bis **80 a & b**, the ball attachment may be preferred due to this problem, depending on the condition of the remaining teeth.

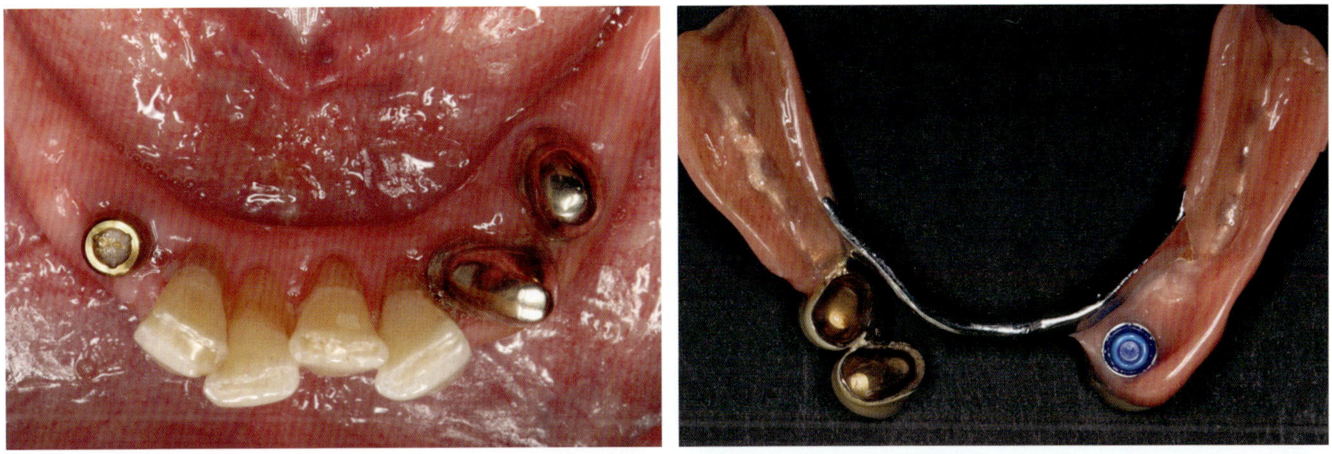

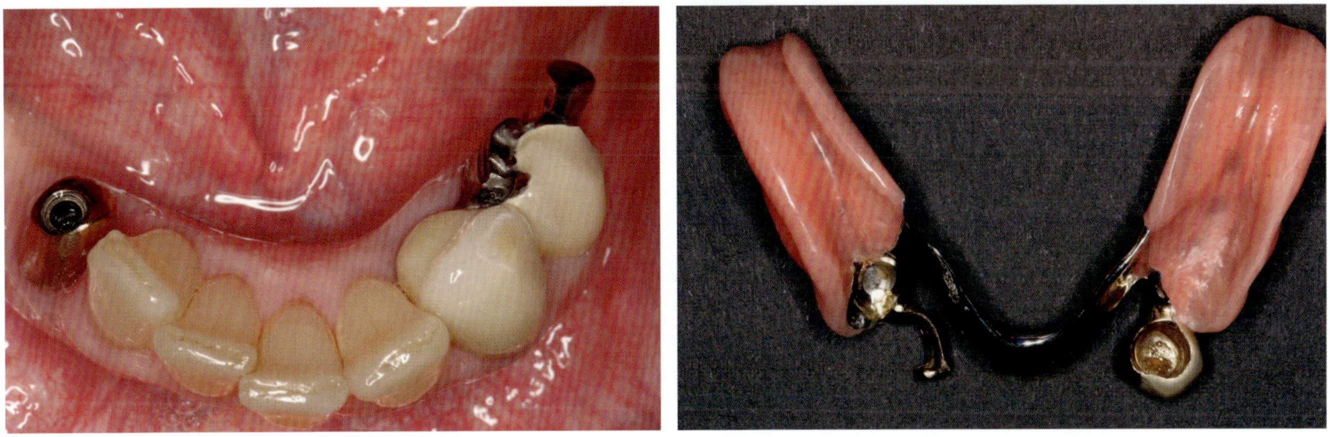

Figs. 79 a & b: Integrated locator in existing denture
Figs. 80 a & b: Integrated telescope in already existing denture

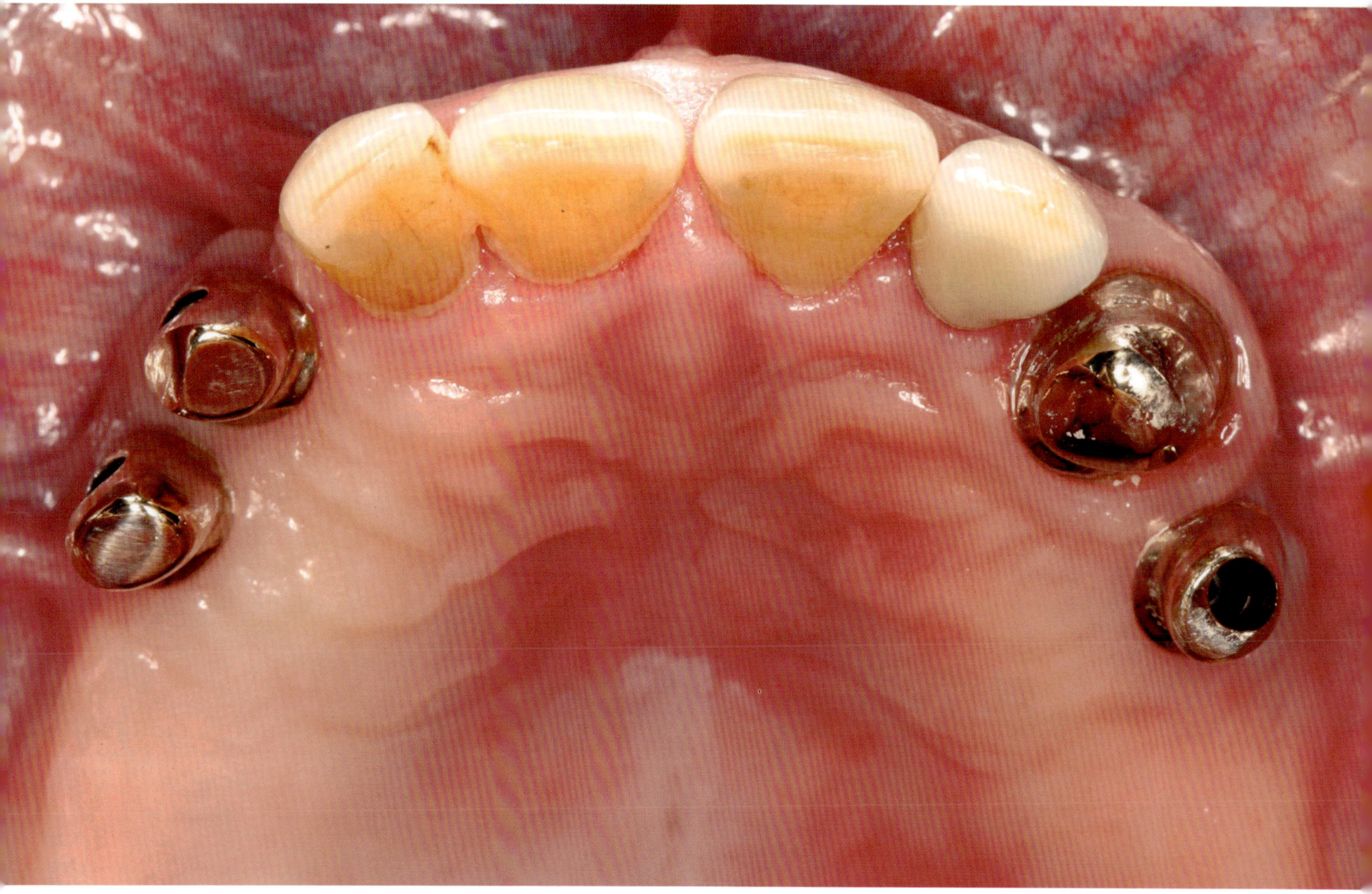

Figs. 81 a & b: Tooth-implant-supported and mucosa-supported suprastructure

Clinical and technical procedure:

Both the implants as well as the natural teeth are restored with telescopic crowns, which are usually manufactured with a 2 - 4° milling angle. In the case of implants, the milled/customized abutment usually takes on the function of the primary part. Unfavorable implant axes can be aligned parallel to the remaining abutments using the inner telescope. The clinical impression is taken in two steps: the impression of the natural teeth is taken first. After that, the impression of the implants is taken in the second step together with the fixation impression of the primary parts using individual trays. This increases the precision of the master cast. Different material and design concepts are described and applied.

Numerous design options are available, ranging from conventional gold castings to milled NPM abutments/primary parts and ceramic primary parts with galvanic or PEEK secondary frameworks. In the author's opinion, the consistent fabrication of

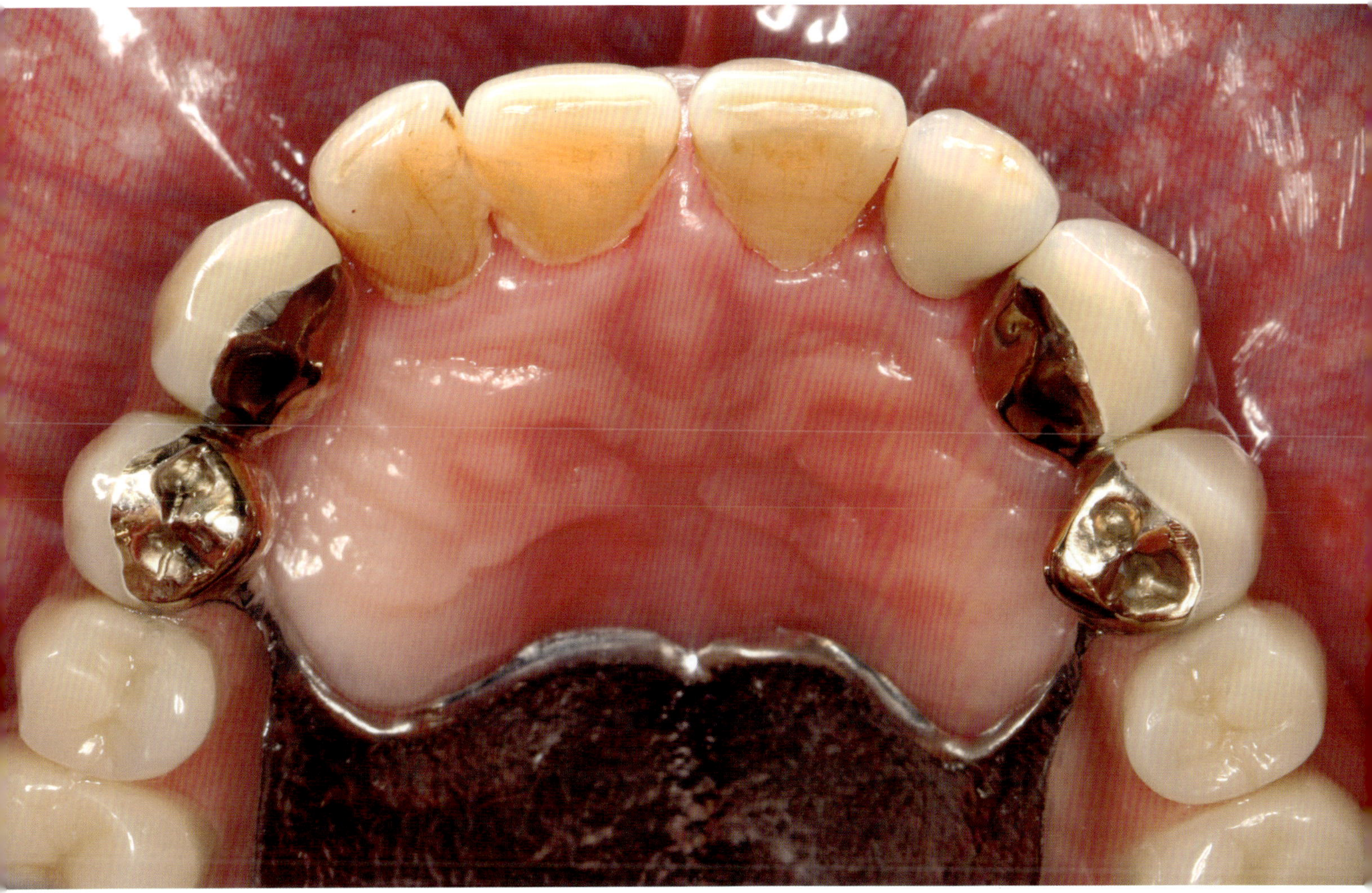

telescopic restorations in the digital workflow, in particular those made of non-precious metal alloys without additional retention aids, has not yet been fully developed.
In principle, the author prefers to use conventionally cast telescopes or thin cast copings (Figs. **81 a & b**), which are bonded in the mouth, instead of secondary elements fabricated by galvanic techniques. Particularly in the case of free-end situations, it has been shown that, due to the pronounced leverage effect of the saddles, the softer alloy of galvanized telescopes is subject to "bending" and increased abrasion, even when closely embraced by the model casting. This may result in a loss of retention of the suprastructure. It is therefore recommended that galvanotelescopes be used primarily where polygonal support is available.

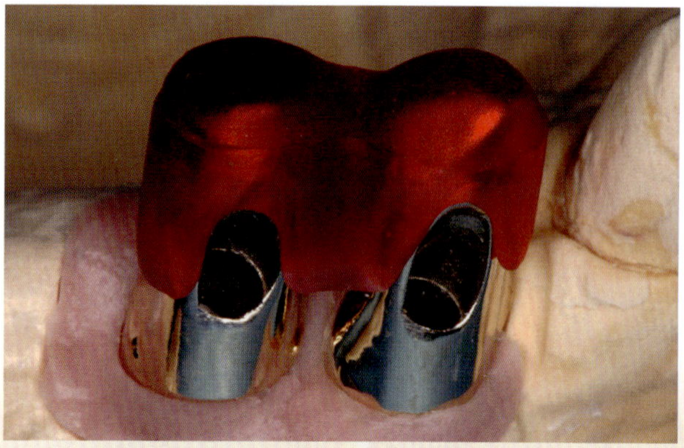

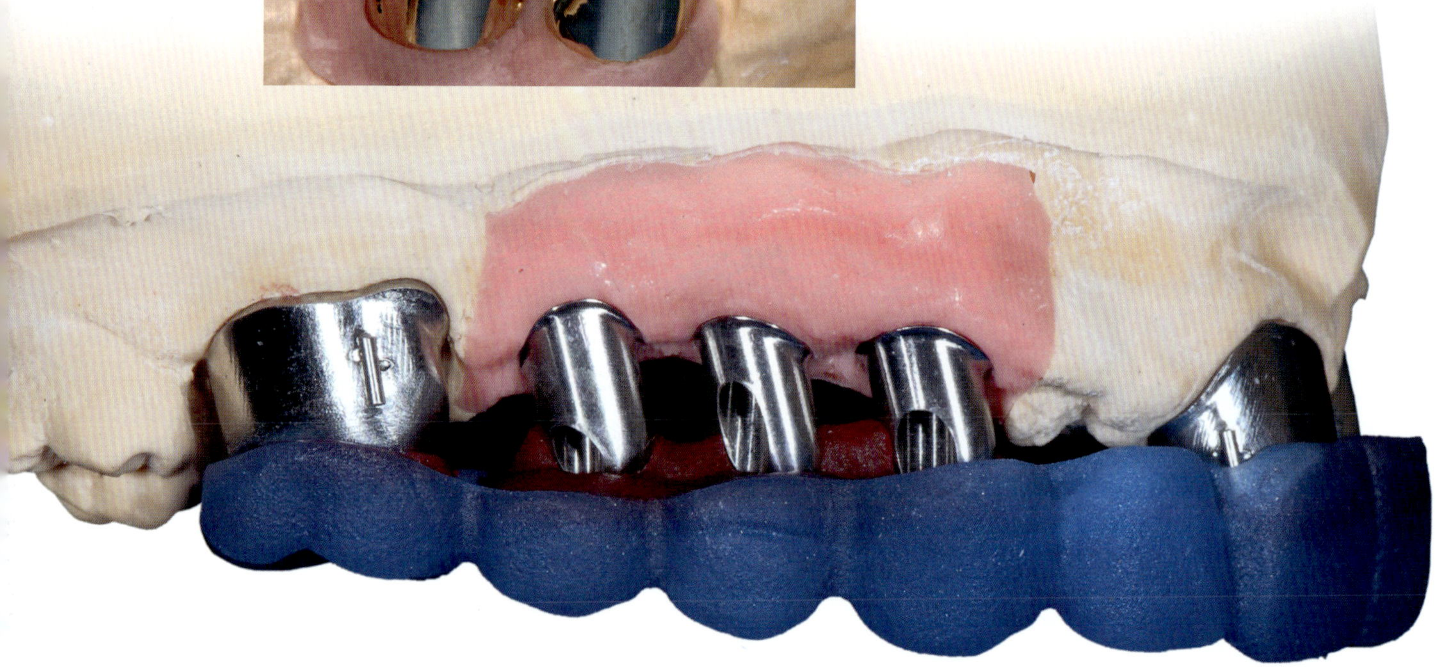

Figs. 82 a & b: Insertion key for exact, rotationfree abutment placement

The fact that every implant system has a certain degree of micromovement in its implant-abutment connection [95] can lead to inaccuracies in the fit and to tension. To ensure a comparable abutment position in the mouth and on the model, at least one insertion key should always be used for the abutments. (Figs. **82 a & b**). Unlike a tooth, an implant is not able to yield and is therefore usually responsible for problems with the fit.

This circumstance can be taken into account as an option to the conventional fabrication of the secondary framework, by the secondary parts on the implants being bonded intraorally during such work.
Strictly speaking, the primary parts should not be unscrewed again. When consistently working in accordance with the “Passive Fit”, the abutments, which are fixed with a final torque, remain in the mouth. This approach is laborious, as it usually requires a new temporary solution or “travel dentures”.

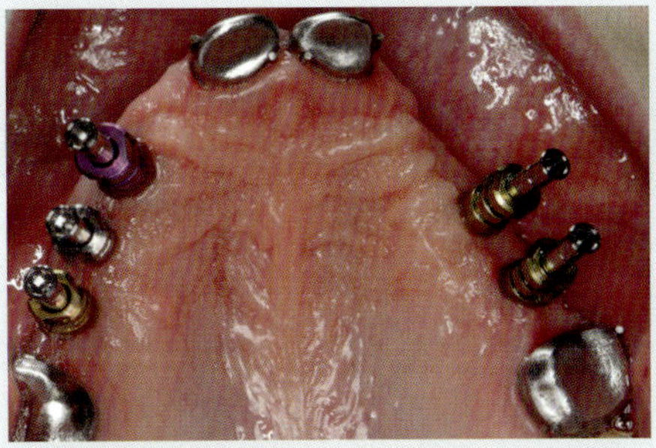

Fig. 83: Fixation impression over milled NPM primary parts

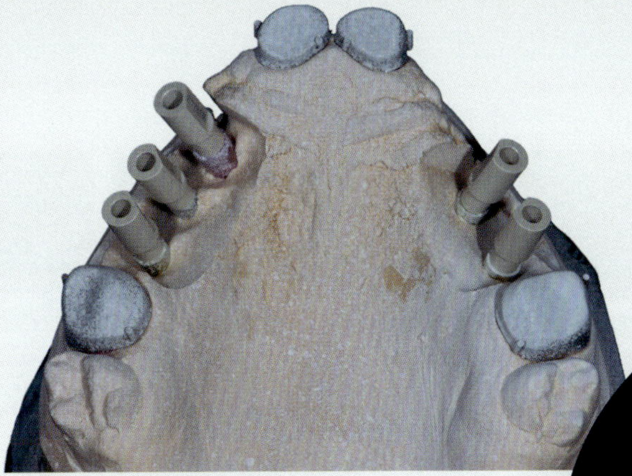

Fig. 84: Model before the scan (photo: Ralf Ommerborn)

Documented patient case (limited to the prosthetic restoration): consistent "Passive Fit" in tooth-/implant-supported telescopic bridge.

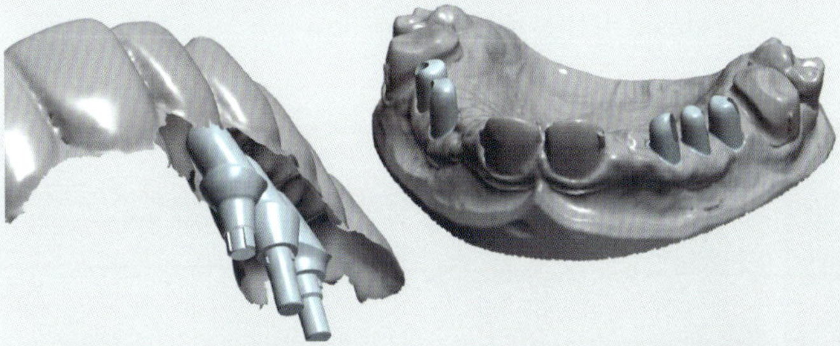

Figs. 85 a & b: Planned customized NPM CAD/CAM abutments

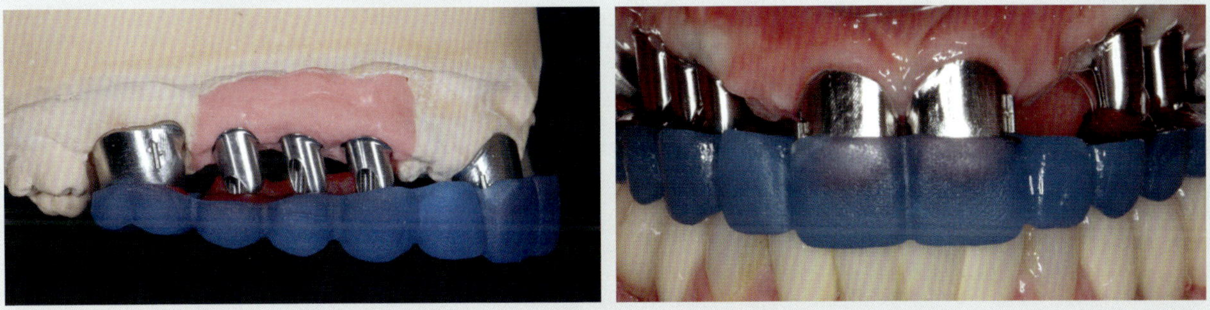

Fig. 86 a & b: Abutment try-in and second bite registration

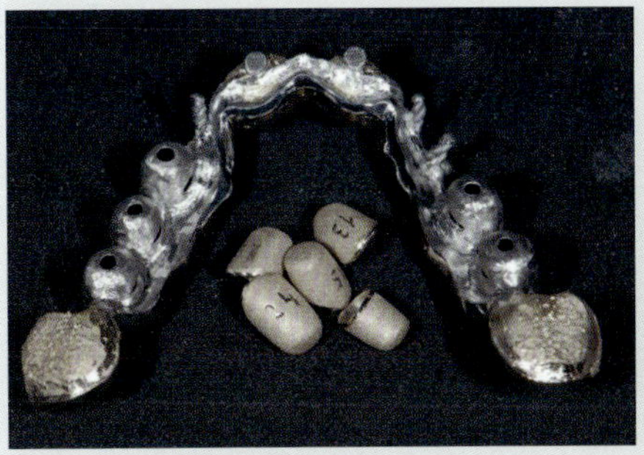

Fig. 87: Secondary parts and CoCr-cast before bonding

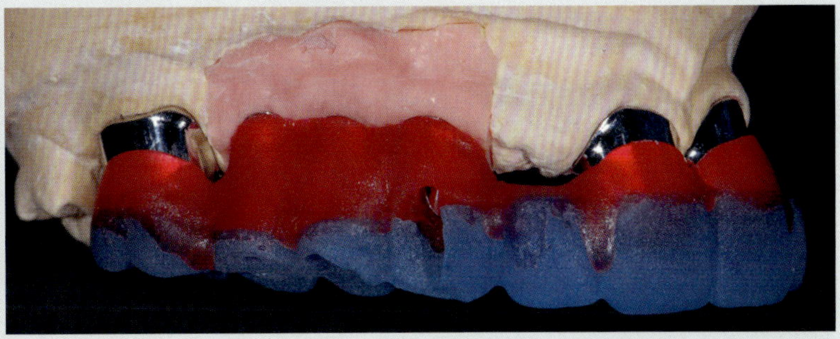

Fig. 88: Insertion key for the abutments/primary parts

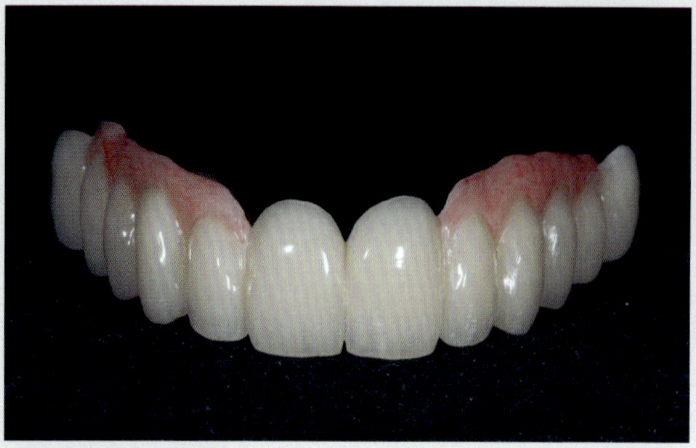

Fig. 89: Provisional denture for restoration after insertion of the primary parts

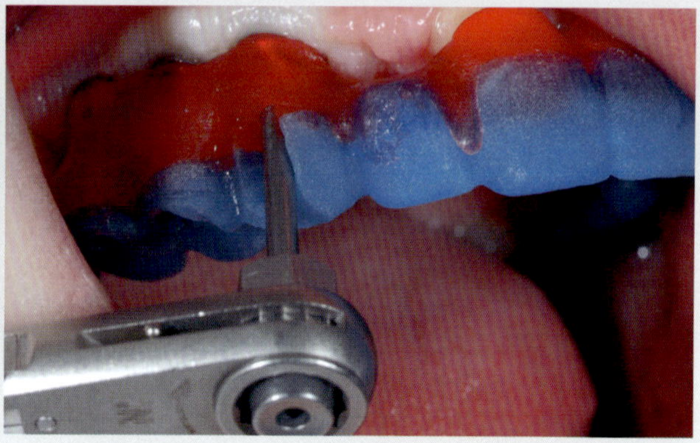

Fig. 90: Final fixation of the abutments (these remain in the mouth from now on)

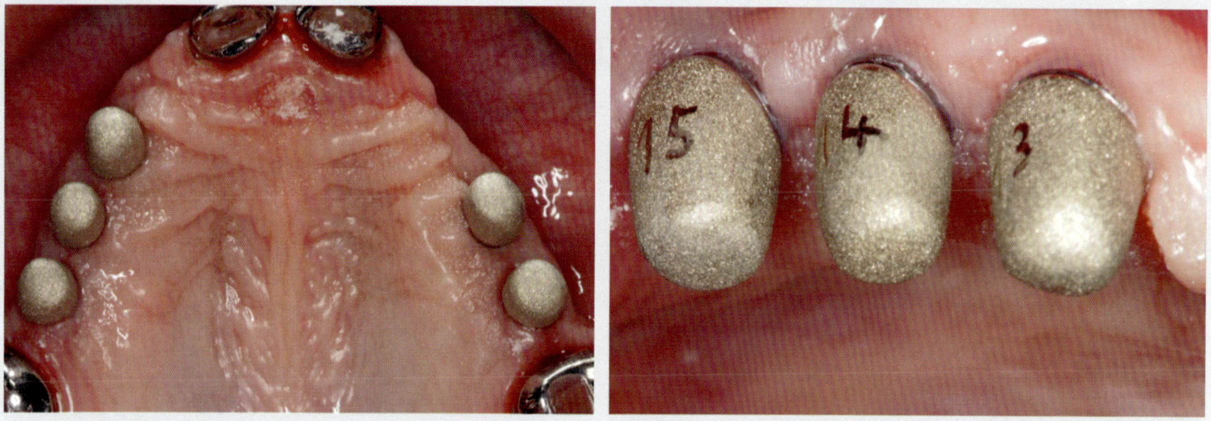

Figs. 91 a & b: Insertion of the thin casted secondary parts

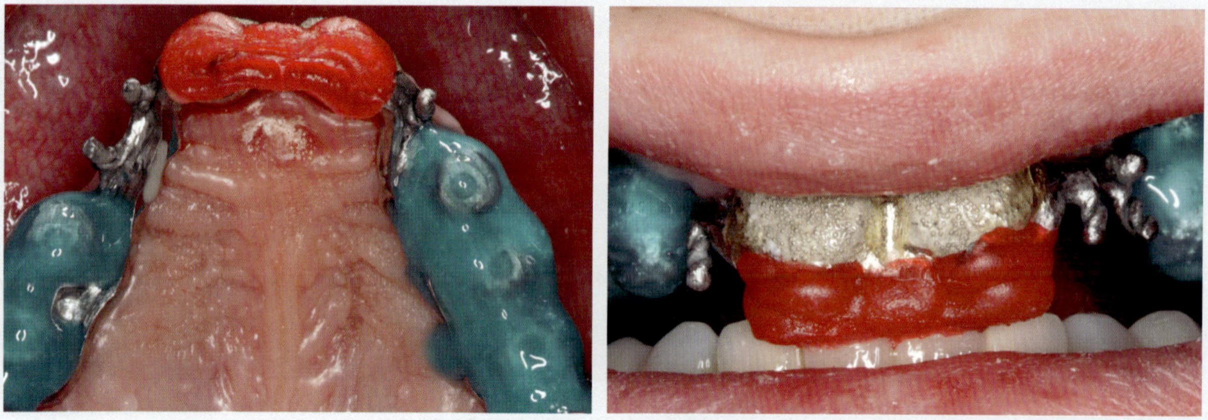

Figs. 92 a & b: Intraoral bonding of the secondary parts with metal casting under masticatory load

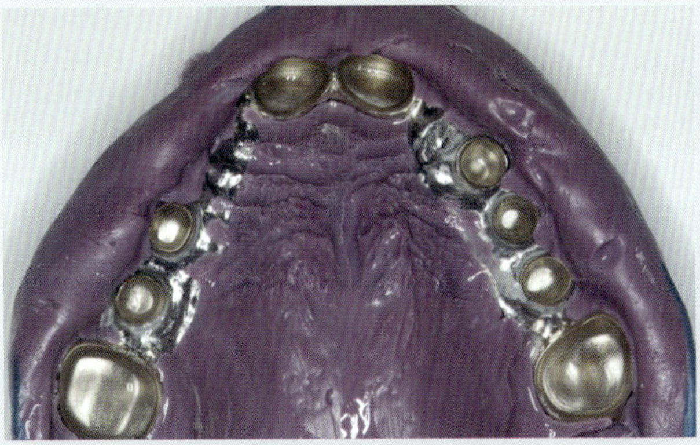

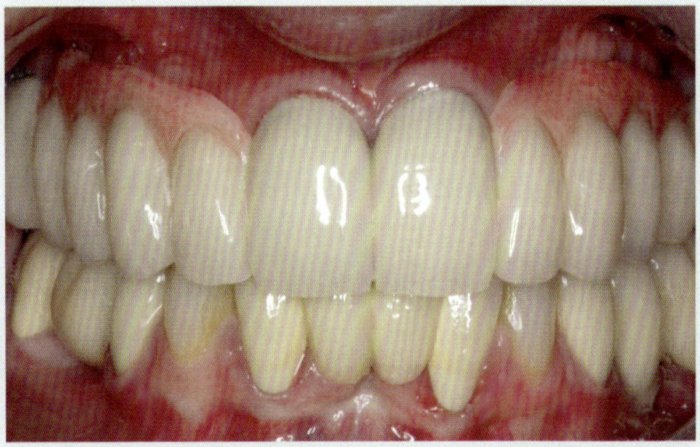

Fig. 93: Over-impression with polyether impression material

Fig. 94: Integrated provisional denture

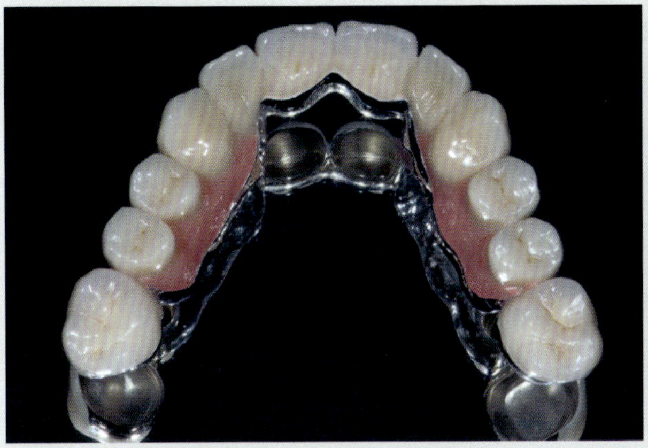

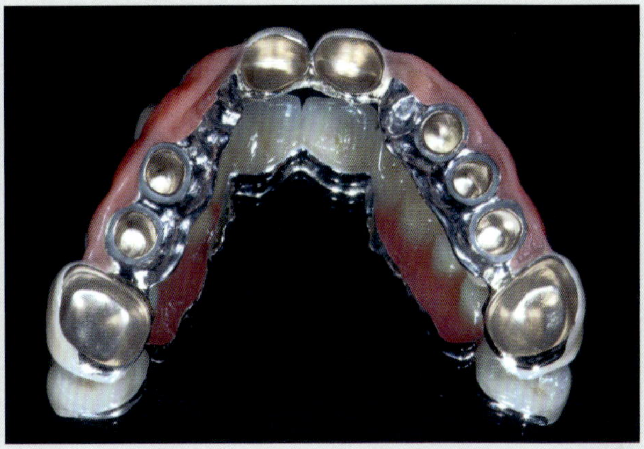

Figs. 95 a & b: Completed restoration

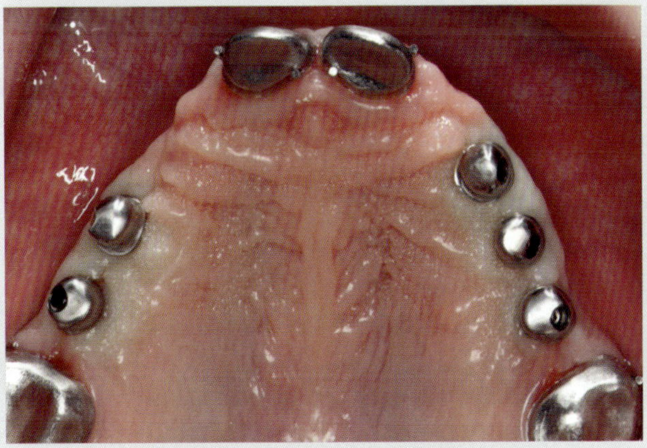

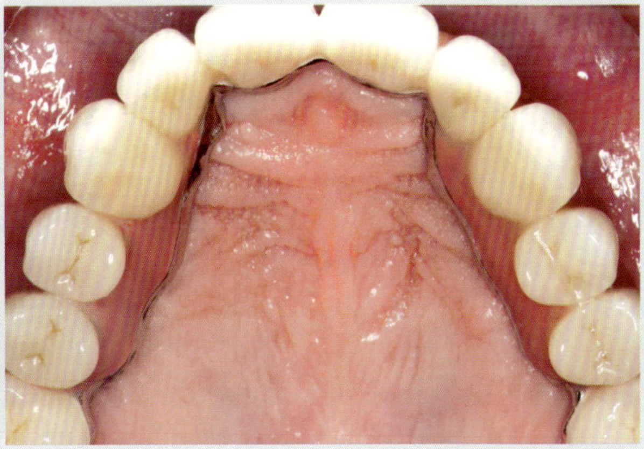

Figs. 96 a & b: Integrated telescopic bridge

2

2.5.

Provisional restoration of the partially or fully edentulous jaws

If the reduced or edentulous jaw lacks natural abutment teeth for temporary support, then inserting temporary implants for anchoring is an option. These transitional implants are immediately loaded with the provisional denture, thus enabling the least possible load on the augmented or implanted jaw sections. This is particularly important in situations where extensive augmentation has taken place, which should be kept as load-free as possible. A prerequisite for the insertion of interim implants is good bone quality, i.e. ideally cortical anchoring. If possible, the vertical bone height should not fall below 10 mm in this case either [96]. In principle, care must be taken not to restrict the position of the definitively planned implants, in other words, to maintain a sufficient distance from the planned implant position.

WIf the described conditions are not given and there is still sufficient residual dentition, another option is to bridge the healing time or temporary phase by leaving extraction-worthy residual abutment teeth (Figs. **97a & b**). This option is generally given if teeth in the periodontally damaged dentition do not cause any discomfort despite an increased degree of loosening and can therefore be left temporarily as abutments.

This form of treatment is suitable in particular if the teeth have previously been restored with crowns or bridges. During the planning phase, it must be determined which teeth are best suited for this purpose in terms of statics, distribution and periodontal condition. With this procedure, consistent anti-infective therapy of the remaining teeth with prior periodontal damage is essential to counteract the risk of possible microbial cross-infection between teeth and implants. The teeth are left in place until temporary or final restoration of the implants is performed. The basal portion of the provisional bridges should be fabricated of plastic – particularly if metal reinforcement is present – to be able to work on or modify the pontics, for example, for soft tissue contouring, but also after implant disclosure.

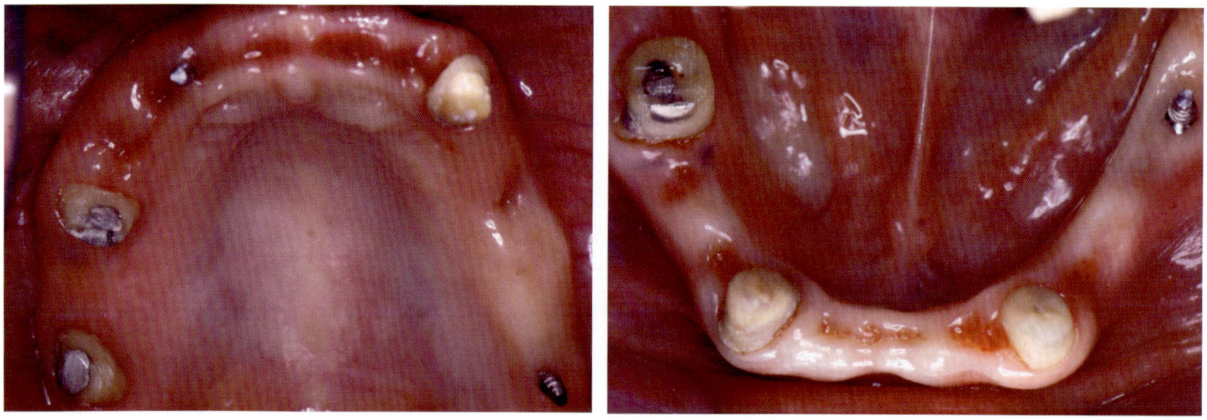

Figs. 97 a & b: Provisional implants and temporarily preserved residual abutment teeth to support a fixed temporary restoration

2.6.

Practical tips for preventing and managing complications

- Patients with loosened prosthetic screws should be treated quickly to avoid damaging the internal thread of the implant. The initial measure for a loosened abutment of a cemented crown that cannot be removed is “trepanation” finding the screw access.

- Any parts remaining in the implant after a screw fracture can, provided there is a certain degree of loosening, simply be removed with a dental probe. To do this, the tip is placed slightly eccentrically on the fragment and then turned continuously in an anticlockwise direction. A system-specific “rescue set” must be used for firmly lodged fragments.

- The prosthesis ratchets should be regularly maintained and checked. Otherwise, especially with those that have a kinking mechanism when the torque is set, there is a risk that the torque acting on the screw is actually significantly higher than assumed.

- In telescopic restorations on teeth and implants, generally the implants cause inaccuracies of fit or “jamming” of the secondary restoration (see explanation on page 56). In this case, the abutments should therefore also be inserted with insertion keys - if possible - or the secondary parts can be bonded intraorally to the metal cast framework in the context of a “Passive Fit”.

- In the author's opinion, electroformed secondary copings should not be used in tooth-implant- supported and mucosa-supported partial dentures with a free-end saddle, as there is a high risk of successive retention loss. The risk is significantly lower with polygonal abutment

- distribution. Thin cast copings generally represent an interesting alternative.

- Insertion keys can also be helpful for easier positioning in the case of deep subgingival implant shoulders during abutment or framework try-ins.

- In the posterior region, hybrid or titanium abutments should be given preference over all-ceramic abutments for fixed cemented restorations, as there is a greater risk of fracture in the area of the inner connection or the anti-rotation lock.

- The decision on the material for the superstructure should take into account both functional and individual circumstances. For example, on rigid implants, the risk of chipping is even greater with veneered zirconia ceramics than on natural teeth.

- Attention should also be paid to the emergence profile in the posterior region. Saddle-shaped contacts of the crowns around the implant neck must be avoided at all costs to prevent limited cleanability as well as the risk of inflammatory peri-implant processes.

- In the case of screw-retained single crowns in the posterior region, implant angulation or possible tilting of the adjacent teeth can, under certain circumstances, make it difficult or even impossible to create long-term sufficient proximal contacts. In such situations, it is therefore occasionally advisable to favor cementation on an appropriately angled abutment.

2.7.
Conclusion

In particular, a significantly reduced and possibly periodontally damaged residual dentition presents the clinician with numerous questions regarding prosthetic planning: fixed or removable restoration? Which teeth are worth preserving and how can they be integrated into a comprehensive implant-based restoration?
Removable restorations using double crowns are particularly suitable for older patients and are certainly a good alternative to fixed restorations. The insertion of implants as “strategic abutments" optimizes the denture statics and, due to better support, load distribution and secondary splinting, can in some cases even improve the prognosis for periodontally damaged remaining abutment teeth that are worth preserving. Cleanability is better than with fixed dentures. Further advantages are the ability to expand, a usually less extensive surgical procedure as well as the option of incorporating additional abutments at a later date. In the author's opinion, older patients who have been accustomed to a removable restoration for many years should rather not be switched to a fixed implant-supported denture.
Implant-prosthetic concepts, whether fixed or removable, cemented or screw-retained, with or without the integration of natural abutment teeth into the restoration, should generally be planned on a patient-specific basis and should, in particular, take into account the patient's individual risk profile.

3

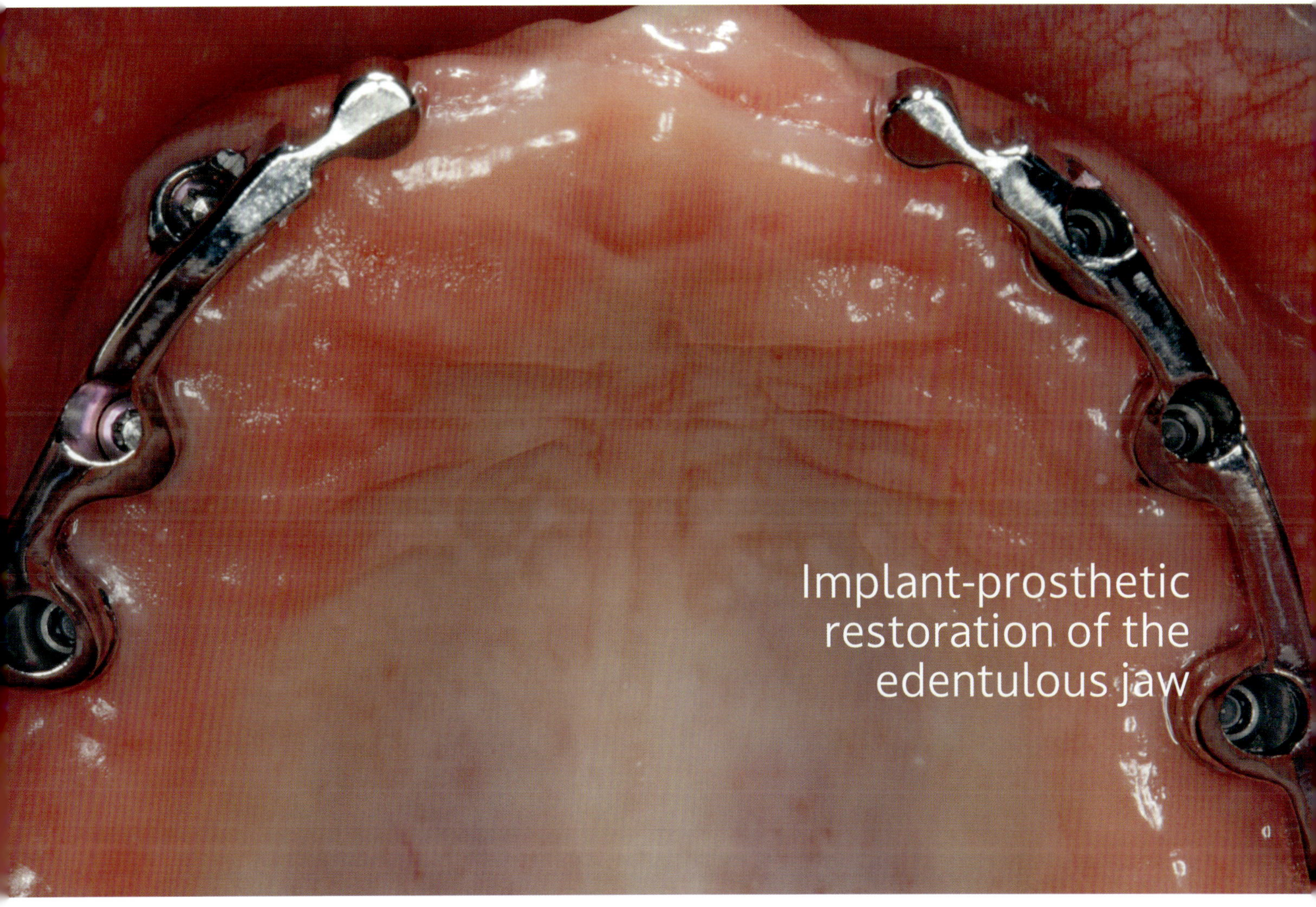

Implant-prosthetic restoration of the edentulous jaw

3.1.
Introduction

As edentulous patients are often of advanced age, implant-prosthetic concepts in these cases should also take into account the general aspects of gerontoprosthodontics. For example, the restorations should be designed to be as easy as possible to use to compensate for limited vision and reduced manual dexterity. Furthermore, the restorations should be extendable to allow for prospective planning, particularly in older patients.
Depending on patient-related factors, anatomical initial conditions or the individual treatment goal, both fixed as well as immediate treatment concepts can be realized in the maxilla and mandible in addition to removable restorations. In particular, these restorations often make complex backward planning unavoidable and place high demands on planning, implant position and prosthetic restoration.

3.2.
Diagnostics and planning

In terms of available bone in the edentulous jaw, the duration of edentulism and the degree of atrophy must first be determined. (Figs. **98a & b**). Even in the case of residual dentition, the condition of the bony foundation should be checked. The qualitative and quantitative classification was conducted by Lekholm and Zarb [99] and is shown in Figures **99** to **100**.

The form of treatment for the edentulous jaw depends not only on the quality and quantity of the remaining bony foundation but also on various extra- and intraoral initial findings (Fig. **101**). With regard to the extraoral situation, particular attention must be paid to the patient's profile, especially the lip support and the vertical relation in the lower third of the face. From the outset, particular attention should also be given to the contour of the smile line.

When **decision making** between fixed or removable dentures, the findings listed on page 66 should be examined and discussed, possibly also by means of a model analysis, in addition to the individual patient-related factors.

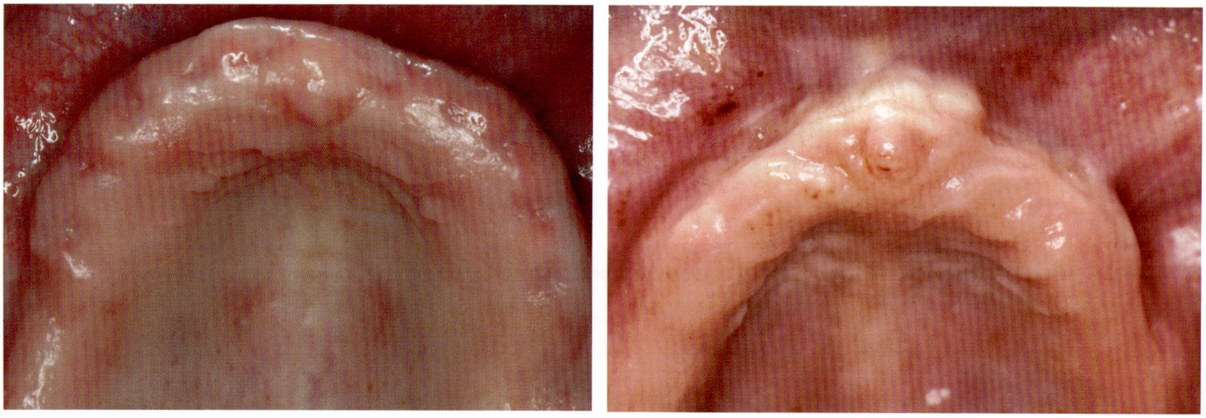

Figs. 98 a & b: Important criterion: duration of edentulism

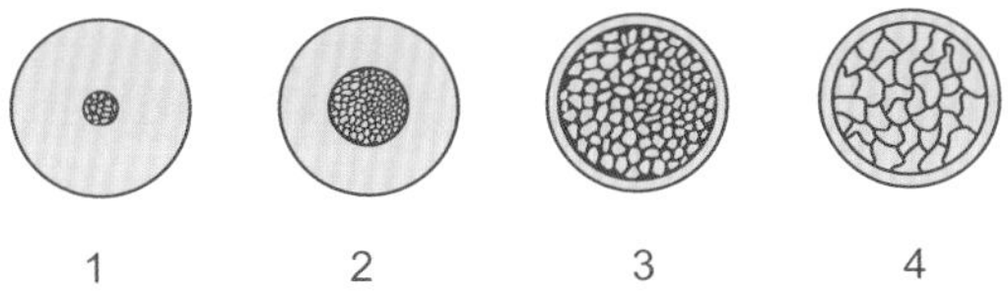

- Type 1 homogenous compact bone
- Type 2 thick cortical bone surrounding dense trabecular bone
- Type 3 thin cortical bone surrounding dense trabecular bone
- Type 4 very thin cortical bone surrounding low-density trabecular bone

Fig. 99: Bone density according to Lekholm and Zarb 1985

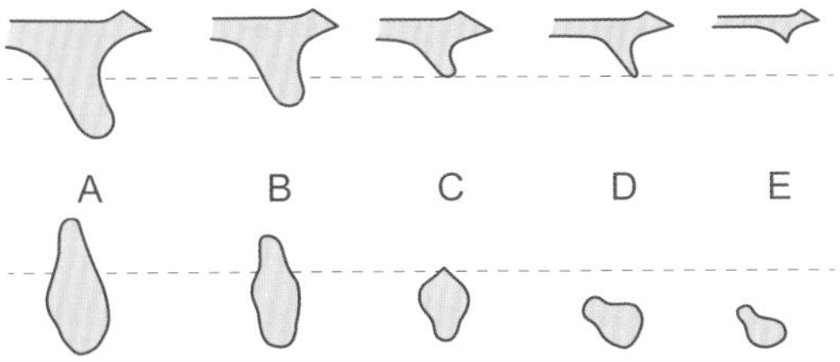

- A: virtually complete alveolar ridge
- B: minor resorption of the alveolar ridge
- C: advanced resorption of the alveolar ridge down to the base of the jaw
- D: initial resorption of the jaw base
- E: considerable resorption of the jaw base

Fig. 100: Degree of atrophy according to Lekholm and Zarb 1985

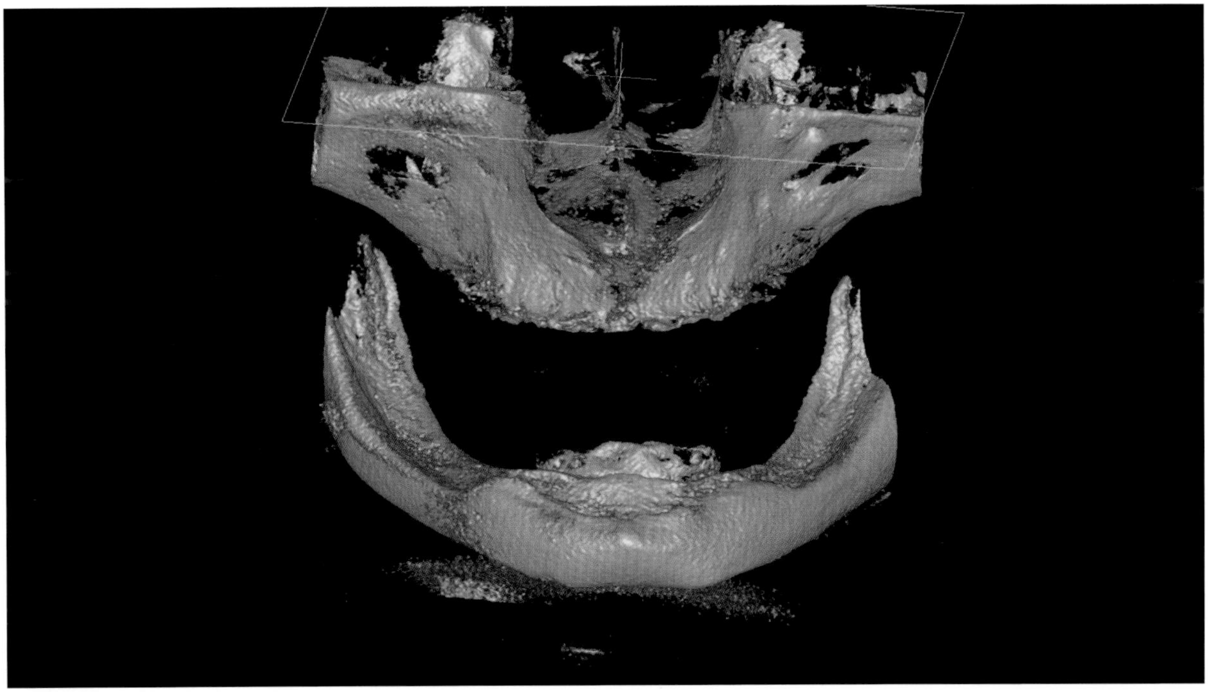

Fig. 101: DVT of highly atrophic edentulous maxilla and mandible

- **Hard and soft tissue morphology:**
  The available bone volume must be consistently clarified radiologically. In particular, a three- dimensional assessment of the compromised bony foundation is useful to be able to plan the further course of treatment predictably. Due to the bony atrophy, there is often an excess of soft tissue with a simultaneously reduced attached gingiva. In some circumstances, a mucogingival correction may be indicated prior to implant placement or in combination with implant surgery.

- **Intermaxillary distance**
  A large interalveolar vertical distance rather indicates the use of removable dentures, as the missing hard and soft tissue can be compensated for by means of the denture base.

- **Skeletal relationship of the upper and lower jaw in the sagittal plane (Angle Class I-III)**
  A fundamental problem in the edentulous jaw is the transversal discrepancy resulting from the centrifugal atrophy in the lower jaw as well as the centripetal resorption in the upper jaw. Edentulous patients with Angle Class II or III relationships tend to be classified as being difficult to treat with fixed implant-supported prosthetic measures. In most cases, restoration with coverdenture constructions is to be given preference and, in the case of extreme discrepancies between the upper and lower jaw, implant placement may sometimes be contraindicated [100]. The problem is that in Class III situations in the lower jaw, the implants usually have to be positioned lingually or tilted for prosthetic reasons. This can lead to a narrowing of the tongue space and to mucogingival problems, as the implants are anchored in the movable part of the floor of mouth mucosa and thus there is very little or no attached gingiva. Restoration of a progenous initial situation may possibly present an indication for three- dimensional presurgical planning and backward planning to accurately predict the position and axial inclination of the implants.

- **Phonetics:**
  Phonetic difficulties can occur after both upper and lower jaw restorations with dentures. Therefore, narrowing of the tongue space should be avoided as far as technically possible. When designing the superstructure, care must also be taken to avoid gaps through which air or saliva could escape.

- **Number of implants:**
  The number of implants generally determines whether a restoration can be designed fixed or removable, although treatment concepts with a reduced number of implants in the upper and lower jaw ("All-on-4") can have a good long-term outcome [101]. The number of implants required depends, among other things, on the planned type of restoration, the bone quality and the implant length. Mandible and maxilla require different planning due to the differing bone morphology. This will be discussed in more detail in the following.

- **Perioral soft tissue support:**
  Even in case of sufficient implants for anchoring a fixed bridge, a cosmetically appealing support of the soft tissue (lip support) can only be achieved by means of removable dentures due to alveolar atrophy. Only here can the often necessary supporting labial shield be designed accordingly. If a fixed restoration is planned and there is an extreme discrepancy between the implant position and the cosmetically necessary position of the labial surfaces of the anterior teeth, the upper lip may no longer be able to slide freely back into the resting position when laughing, or the region around the philtrum and above the upper lip may droop optically. (Figs. **102 – 106**). A so-called esthetic try-in before creating the framework is therefore of particular importance.

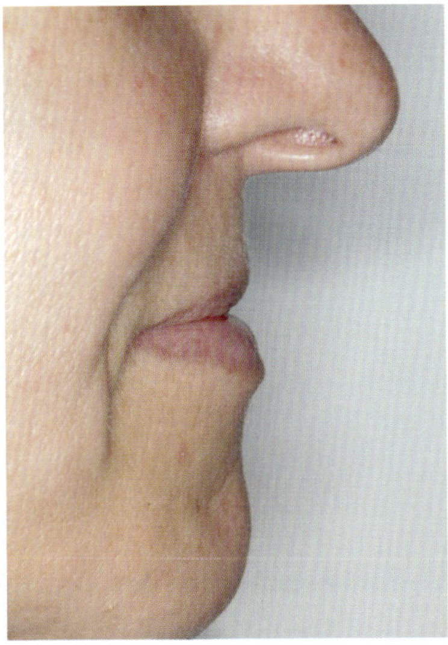

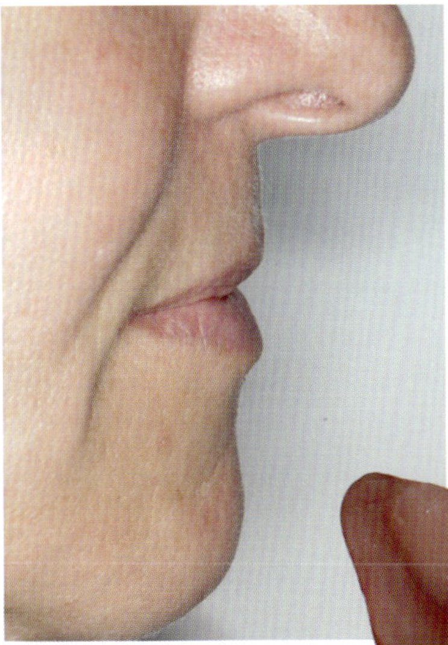

Fig. 102: Female patient with bite template without vestibular shield requesting a fixed bridge restoration

Fig. 103: Female patient with interim prosthesis including labial plastic shield and better support of the extraoral soft tissues

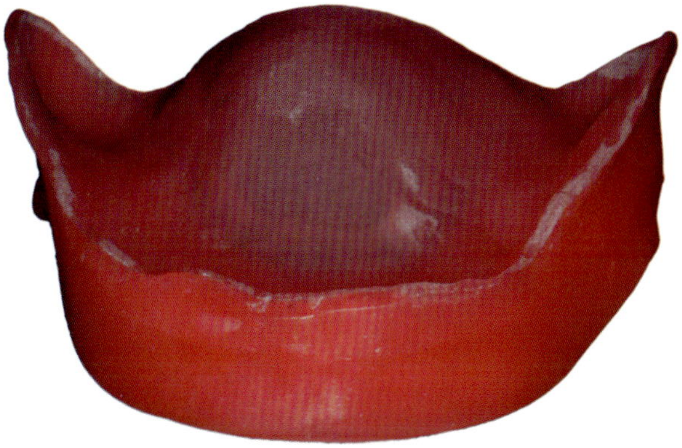

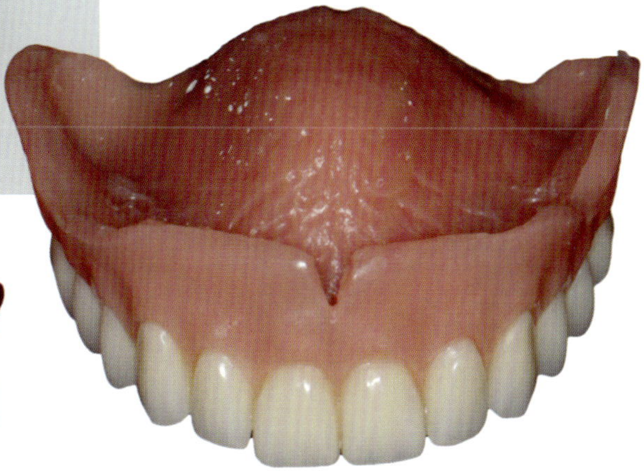

Figs. 104 a & b: Comparison of a bite template (simulating the maximum anterior position of the labial surfaces without alabial shield) and an interim prosthesis

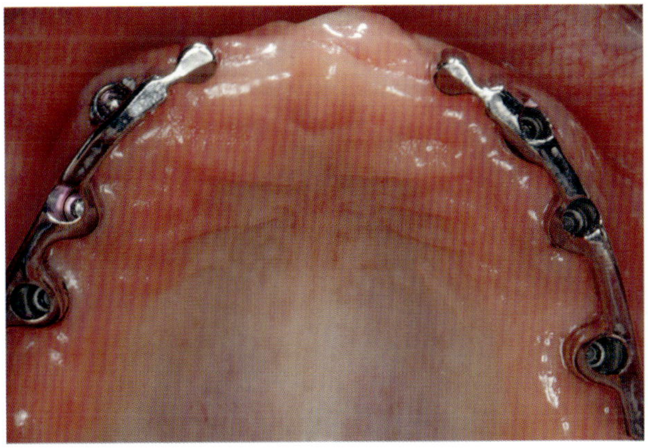

Fig. 105: Divided and milled NPM bar

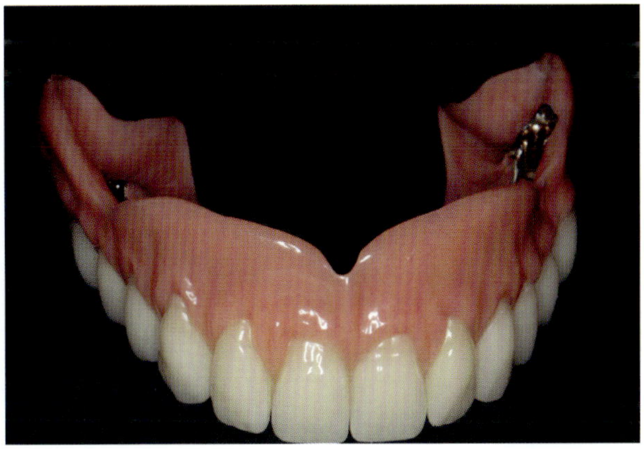

Fig. 106: Removable implant-supported denture with labial shield

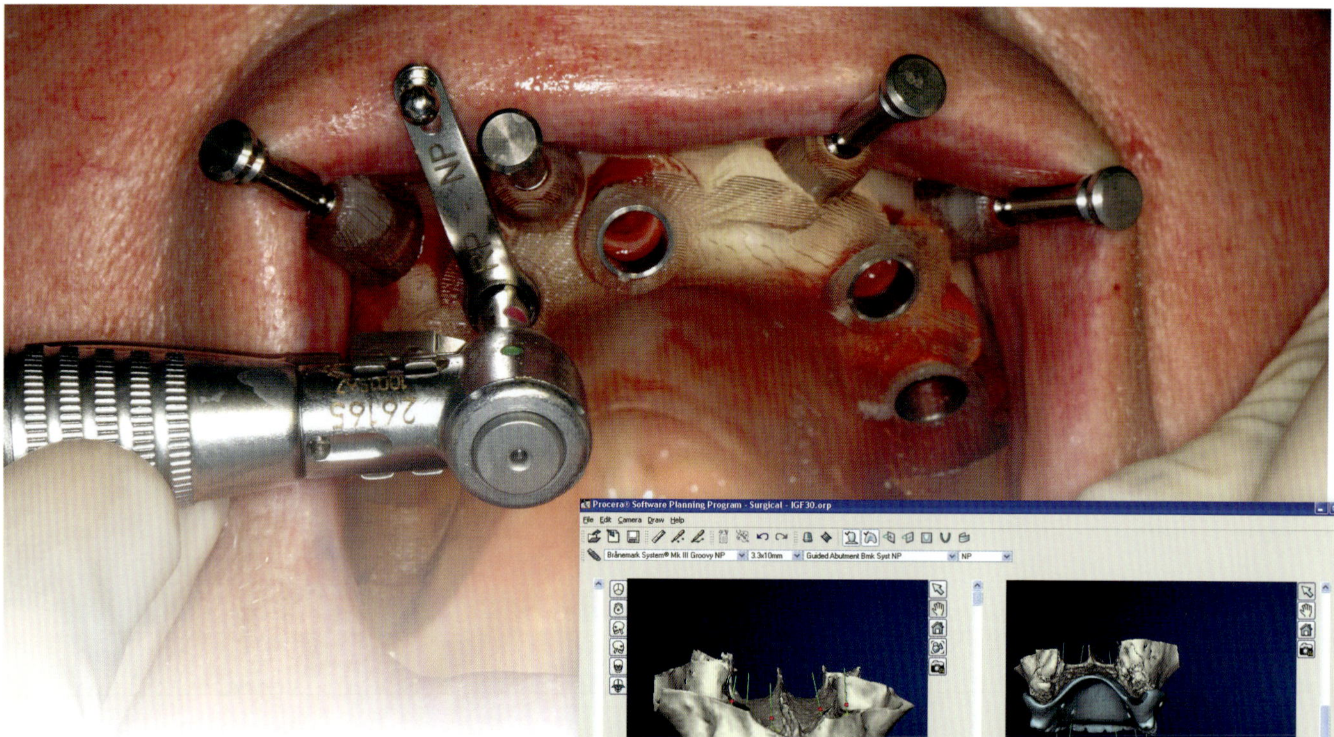

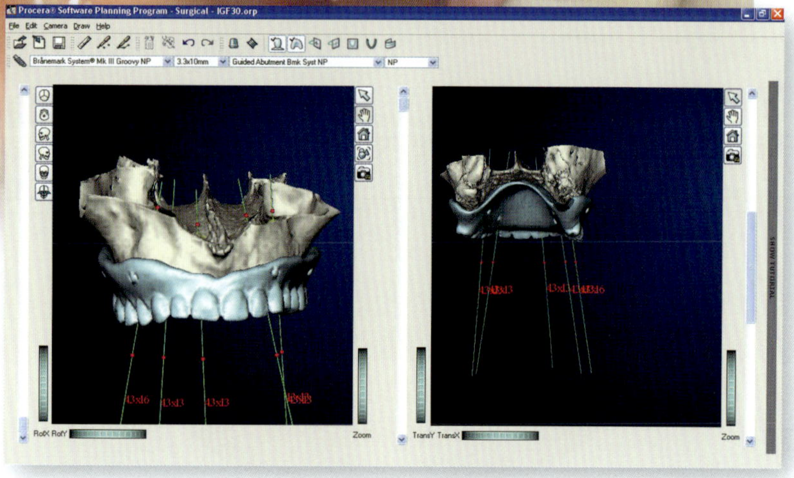

Figs. 107 a & b: Fully guided implant insertion using a surgical guide fixed with anchor pins

In general - particularly with regard to the maxilla - one should never promise the patient fixed restorations too soon. Unless, of course, the above findings or consistent backward planning have been carefully implemented. Even after implant placement, possible malpositioning or implant loss can make it impossible to realize a fixed restorarion. For some time now, three- dimensional diagnostics using CT or digital volume tomography (DVT) have proven to be the most accurate method of planning. Combined with prosthetic planning, the optimal implant position can be determined preoperatively on this basis and transferred during template-guided implant insertion. (Figs. **107 a & b**).

Overall, this leads to a better predictability of the treatment outcome. This also makes it possible to predict the prosthetical outcome of an immediate restoration (see case study at the end of the chapter) [102, 103].

Nevertheless, it should be emphasized that patient satisfaction with removable suprastructures is similarly good, if not occasionally even better, than with fixed restorations [104, 105]. The author tends to favor a removable restoration, especially for older patients, particularly if the patients have been wearing dentures for a longer period of time.

3.3.

Restoration of the edentulous mandible

In the edentulous lmandible, especially in older patients, the resorption processes are usually advanced and therefore the conditions with regard to hard and soft tissue and the relation of the jaws to each other are often not ideal. In particular, this affects the posterior sections of the mandible, so that implants in the severely atrophic mandible can usually only be inserted in the interforaminal region. There, the long-term prognosis is considered to be very good [106]. A lesser degree of atrophy or good bone availability also allows a more posterior implant positioning in principle. With regard to the number of implants, the implant position and the type of suprastructure, a distinction is made between different concepts for the restoration. The nomenclature presented below for the upper and lower jaw is based, in a modified form, on the classification published by Prof. H. Spiekermann in 1990. The treatment concepts 1–4 in the following explain removable and fixed restoration options in the edentulous mandible – from a bar on two implants to fixed restorations with implants also in the posterior mandible.

3.3.1.

Removable restorations in the edentulous mandible

Treatment concept 1
(removable overdenture on two implants)

By placing two implants in the interforaminal region of the edentulous mandible a removable, mucosa-supported, overdenture - implant supported in the anterior region - can be fabricated. This treatment has been shown to reliably improve masticatory function and quality of life in elderly patients over the long term. [107].
The implants can be primarily splinted with a bar. (Figs. **108 a & b**). In this way, retention is shifted to the bar and thus between the implants. In this case, attention should be paid to a rotation option for the bar framework; rigid connections, e.g. via a bar attachment, are not recommended.

The correct design of the bar is ensured by the appropriate positioning of the implants. The bar should be about 20 mm long and designed straight, so that the implants should be spaced about 22–24 mm apart.

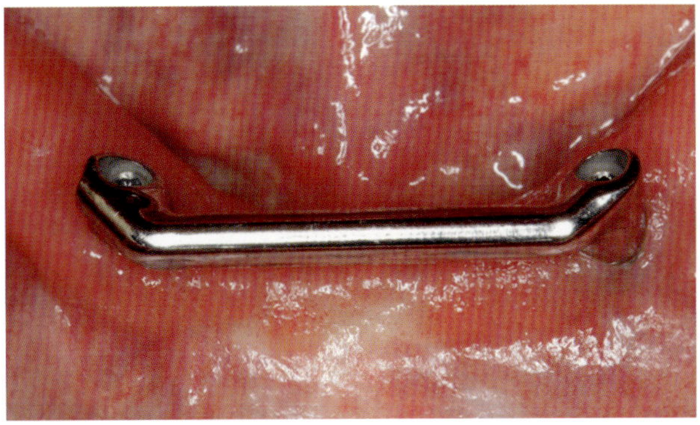

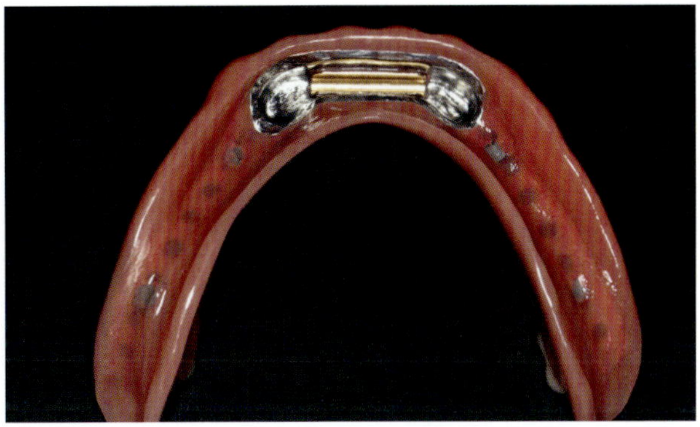

Figs. 108 a & b: Dolder bar and bar overdenture

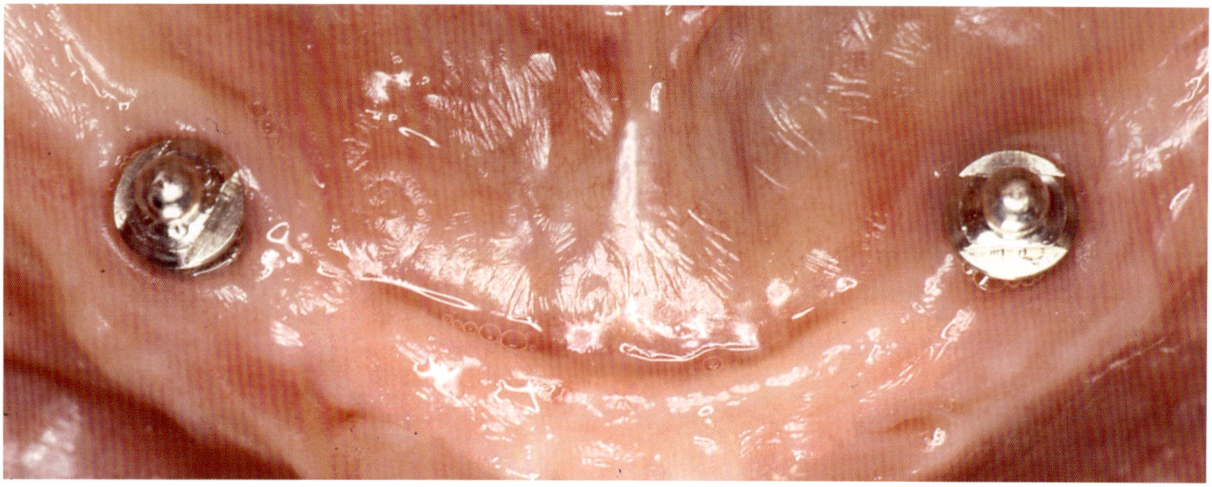

Fig. 109: Ball abutments

Bars that are too short result in reduced retention of the dentures, whereas bars that are too far lingual lead to functional and phonetic restrictions.

As an alternative to bar designs, restoration with individual anchoring systems can be considered. These include, for example, telescopes, ball abutment systems (Fig. **109**), Locators or magnets. The use of Locator systems is a more cost-effective solution that can also be incorporated into existing dentures in certain circumstances. The use of Locators or ball abutments may also be appropriate if the distance between the implants is too great or their position in relation to each other forms a diagonal, thus rendering a restoration using a bar impractical. A bar design may also be contraindicated for very pointed alveolar ridges.
For the sake of completeness, the optional restoration concepts with a central implant [108] or three implants [109] in the anterior edentulous mandible should be mentioned. From the author's point of view, the central implant in particular can cause problems, as the mobility of the soft tissue and muscle attachments are particularlyhigh in this anatomical region.

Treatment concept 2 (removable overdenture on four interforaminal implants)

The entire interforaminal area is utilized here by placing four implants at approximately equal distances from each other. In doing so, the two terminal implants must have a safety distance of 5 mm to the mental foramina. For the sake of clarity and to make safe use of the entire area, the foramina must be visualized intraoperatively.
In the concept with four implants, the overdenture is also designed as a coverdenture prosthesis, i.e. as a removable, mucosa-supported, implant-supported restoration. As anchorage elements for the prosthesis, implants can be restored using bars with or without attachments, telescopic crowns, ball abutments, or Locators [110] (Figs. **110 a & b**).
The bars we use most often these days are usually CAD/CAM-manufactured, parallel-milled non-precious metal bars [111]. They have largely replaced cast gold bars and can be fabricated with or without a distal extension or distal attachment, such as a GSP attachment (groove-shoulder-pin attachment).

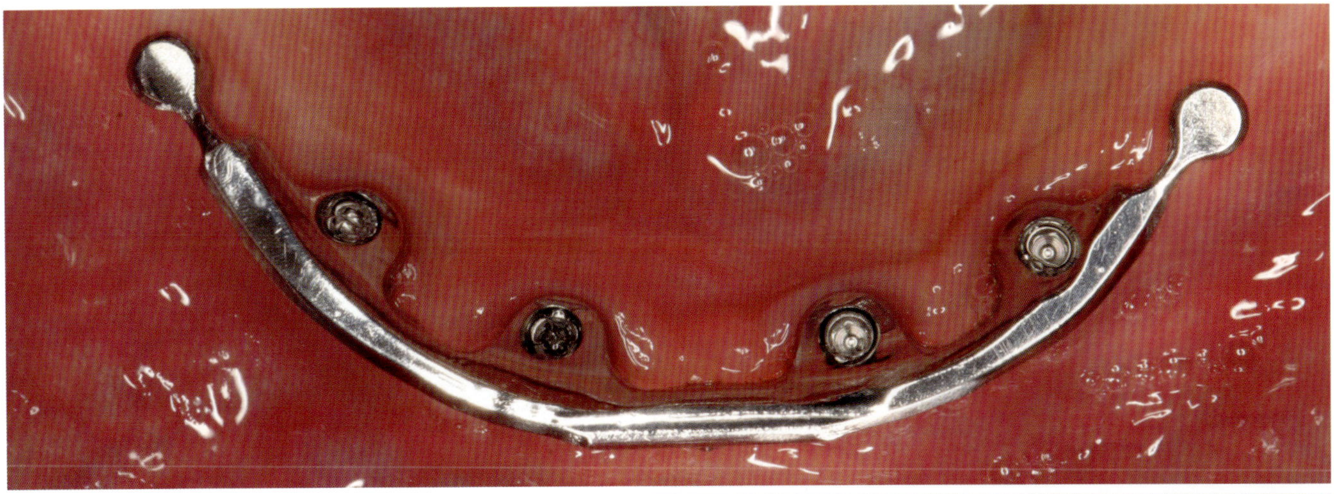

The secure fixation of the removeable denture part is ensured by the use of several bar matrices and/or retaining elements of sufficient length, whereby, in contrast to treatment concept 1, the suprastructure can no longer rotate around the bar. These retaining elements can be made of plastic or gold and should be anchored interchangeably in the secondary structure.

In principle, the overdenture can be fabricated as an anterior implant-supported and posterior mucosa-supported prosthesis or as a fully implant-supported restoration.
If the distance between the anterior and posterior implants is sufficiently large and material-related aspects are taken into account, a long extension bar can be fabricated and the prosthesis can potentially be designed to be fully implant-supported. (Figs. **111a & b**). A fully implant-supported telescopic bridge can also be realized in cases of shortened dental arches.

As a matter of principle, a bar extension should not be longer than the distance between the anterior and posterior anchoring element [112].

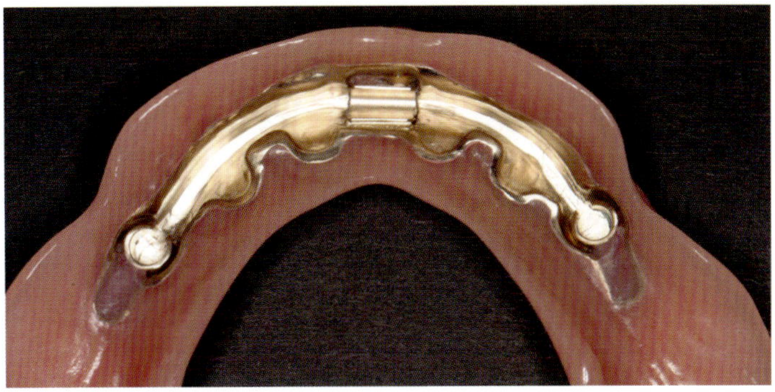

Figs. 110 a & b: Milled NPM bar with terminal attachments and gold matrix in the denture

This is not possible with a frontally flattened jaw arch, if the teeth are to be positioned up to the second molar, additional support must be provided via the mucosa. When four or even five interforaminal implants are positioned closely together, distal extensions can be used effectively as additional retentions. In these cases, the prosthesis must nonetheless be designed with mucosal support in the distal area. Even if appropriately dimensioned, parallel-milled non-precious metal bars are clearly superior to gold bars in terms of stability, the conventional design principles should still be taken into account – especially with regard to the load on the terminal implants.

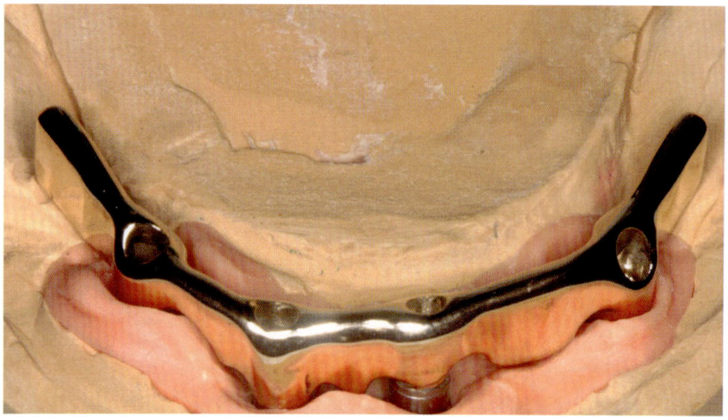
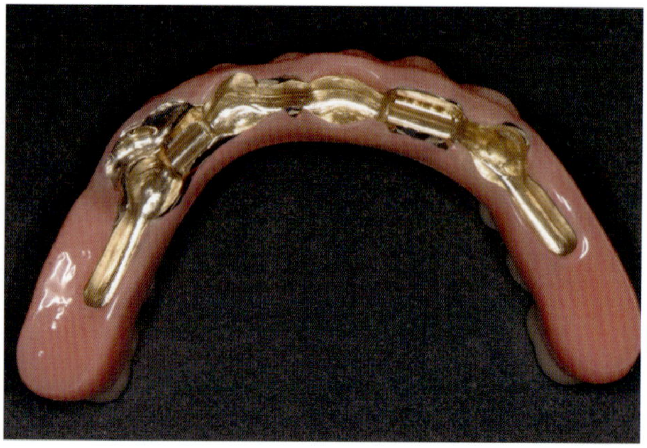

Figs. 111 a & b: Fully implant-supported removable denture on a cast extension bar

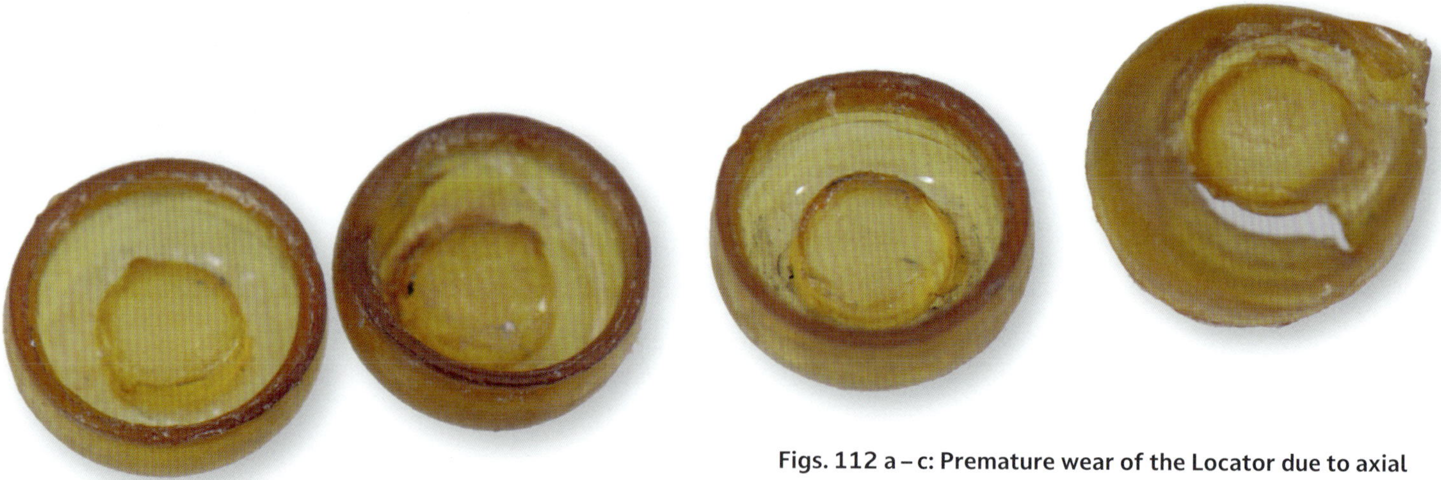

Figs. 112 a – c: Premature wear of the Locator due to axial divergence of the implants (images: Volker Weber)

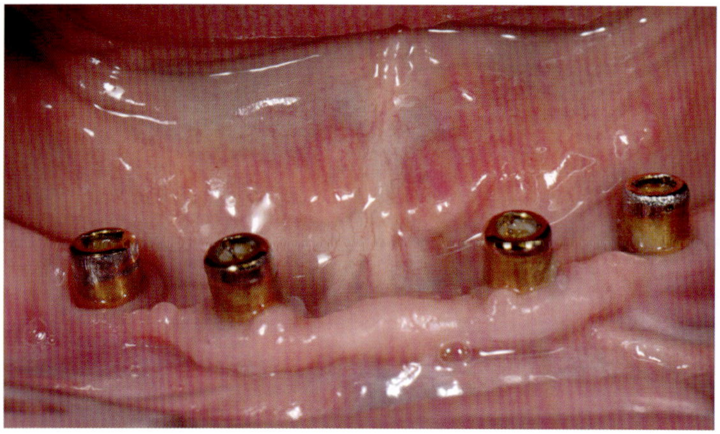
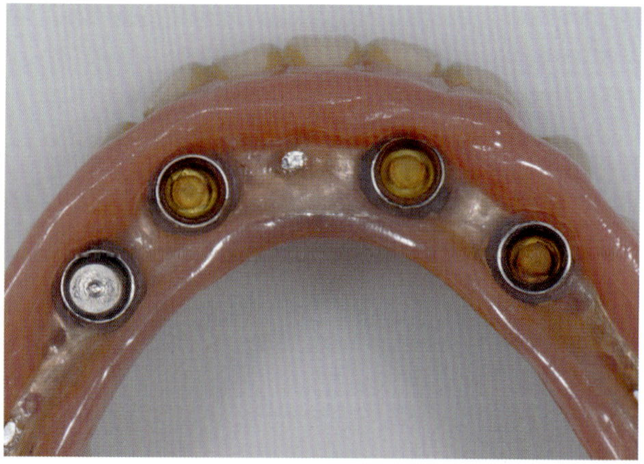

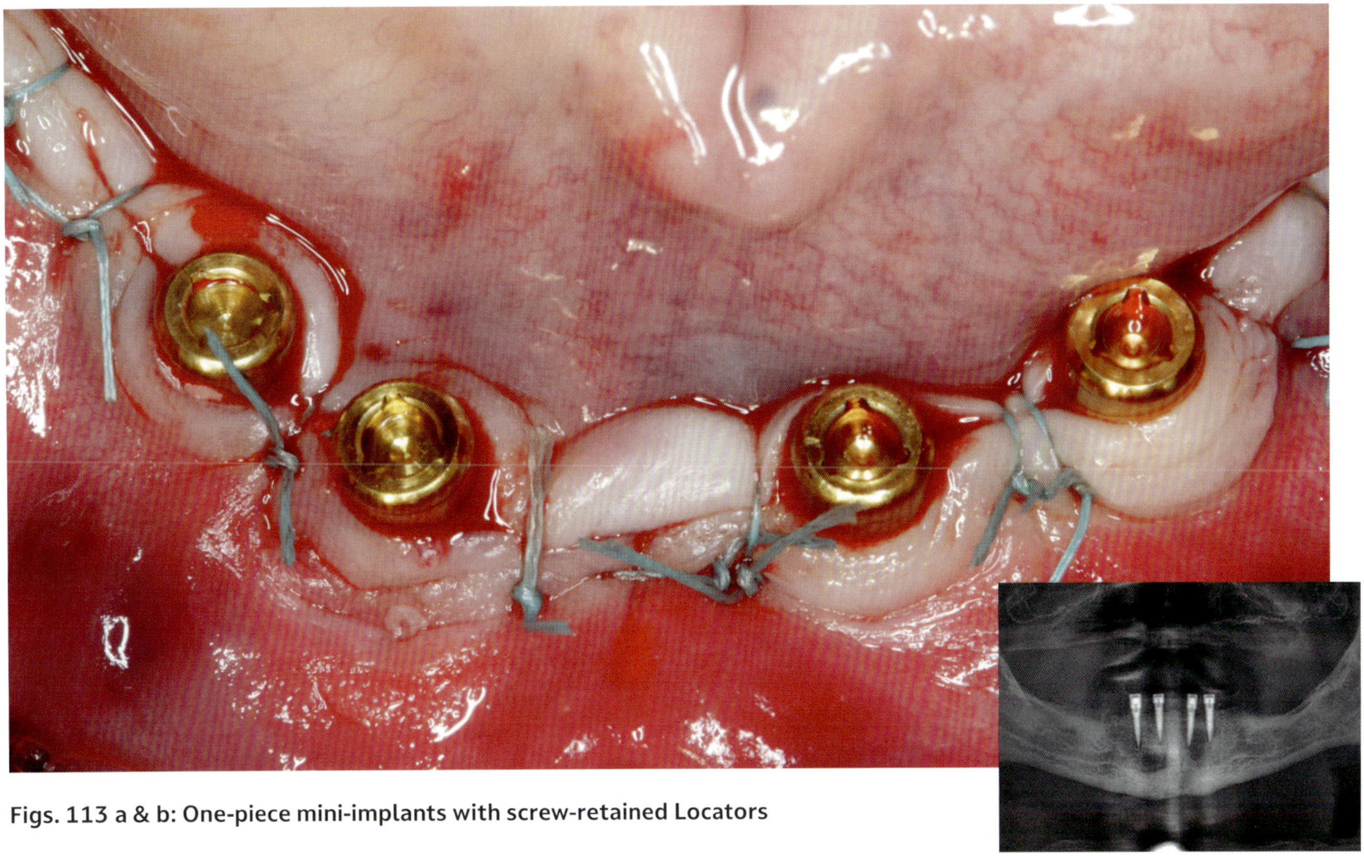

Figs. 113 a & b: One-piece mini-implants with screw-retained Locators

An alternative restoration option for the interforaminal implants is the telescopic prosthesis. One advantage of this design is the more favorable periodontal hygiene when compared to bars. However, with this type of restoration, major prosthetic complications can be expected with the terminal implants, especially with long mucosa-supported saddles.

A restoration using Locators represents a cost-effective alternative. In this case, however, it is important to ensure that the implants are aligned in parallel to avoid premature wear on the matrices or even their guides (Figs. **112a – c**). New angled Locator systems can circumvent this problem.

In principle, a treatment with removable partial dentures offers the advantage of significantly easier oral hygiene maintenance compared to fixed implant-supported cantilever bridges. This consideration should take priority when older patients are, for example, limited in terms of manual dexterity. A large group of patients seems to be more satisfied with a removable denture than with fixed restoration that require a great deal of care [113].

A narrow interforaminal alveolar ridge, limited economic possibilities or a less invasive surgical treatment approach desired due to the patient's age or medical history also allow mini-implants to be considered as a therapeutic alternative. (Figs. **113 a & b**). The results of clinical follow-up examinations and studies are positive and encouraging [114, 115].

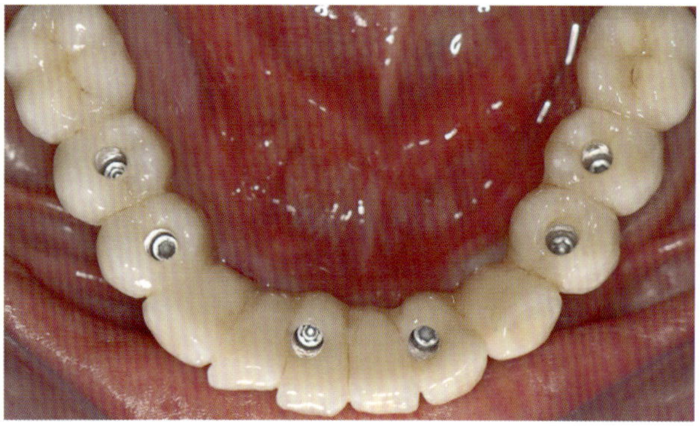

Fig. 114: Cantilever bridge made of zirconium oxide ceramic (image: Patrick Heers)

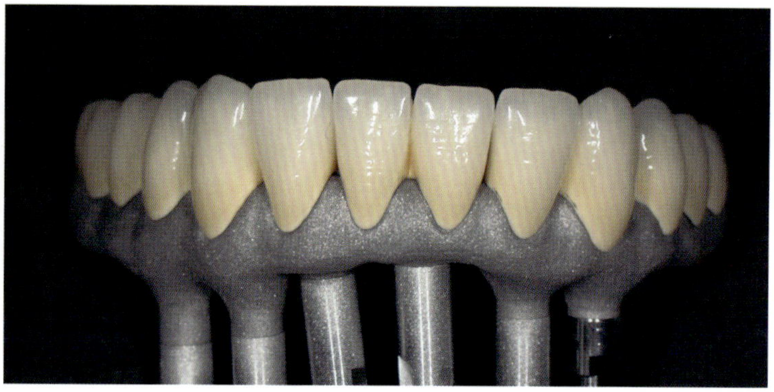

Fig. 115: Cantilever bridge CAD/CAM titanium (image: Oliver Hanisch)

3.3.2.

Fixed restorations in the edentulous mandible

Treatment concept 3 (fixed cantilever bridge on four to five interforaminal placed implants)

This treatment concept describes the restoration using a fixed cantilever bridge on four or five interforaminal placed implants in the edentulous mandible. As a rule, such a suprastructure is screw-retained and can be restored with either metal-ceramic or all-ceramic suprastructures, with or without a mesostructure. (Figs. **114 & 115**).

A conventional bridge restoration with abutments in the area of the first or second molars assumes minimal horizontal and vertical alveolar ridge atrophy posteriorly and necessitates implant placement distal to or superior to the mental foramina. This is rarely the case in the severely atrophic mandible without prior augmentation, so that the design of a fixed restoration as a cantilever bridge is then the norm [116].

If necessary, the restoration can also be performed according to the "All-on-4" concept, if the anatomical conditions allow for implant positioning above the mental foramina. In this case, the distal implants are placed in the apical region with a sufficient safety margin anterior to the mental foramina, but angled approximately 45° posteriorly in the coronal region. This extends the supporting polygon for a fixed cantilever bridge to posterior.
This procedure makes three-dimensional planning or template-guided implant placement advisable to ensure the oblique alignment of the terminal implants while protecting the anatomical neighboring structures. In addition, the "All-on-4" concept also includes immediate restoration of the interforaminally inserted implants using a fixed provisional prosthesis [117].

When fabricating cantilever bridges, care must be taken to ensure that the terminal implants are not overloaded by too long cantilevers and that the framework – especially in the posterior regions – is very stable. (Fig. **116**). in overly delicate suprastructures, overloading can lead to framework fractures and deformations, especially distal to the terminal implant.

As a rule of thumb, the saddles should not be longer than approximately the width of two premolars.

Treatment concept 4 (fixed restoration also with implants in the posterior mandible)

If the anatomical conditions are favorable, it is also possible to place implants in the posterior mandible. In this case, with a favorable distribution of abutments, a restoration with a fixed suprastructure is possible with a number of six to eight implants, taking into account the above-mentioned limiting factors (Figs. **117a & b**). The restoration should consist of at least two bridge segments, preferably several smaller units, for example two to four implants interforaminally and one to two implants posterior to themental foramina on both sides. As severe anatomical restrictions may prevail in the posterior region of the mandible, it may be useful to perform a three-dimensional diagnostic and planning procedure using DVT prior to surgery.

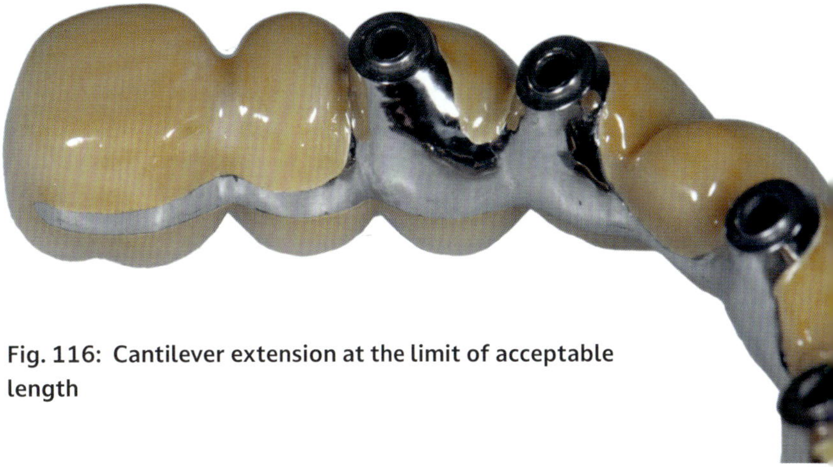

Fig. 116: Cantilever extension at the limit of acceptable length

Due to the deformation of the mandibular splint, there may be isolated cases of a feeling of tension when opening the mouth with fixed, completely splinted restorations in the mandible with implants in the molar region. Therefore, as already mentioned, the construction of multiple bridge segments or several small units should definitely be preferred. These act as “stress breakers” to avoid tension in both the peri- implant bone as well as in the suprastructure. In most cases, it makes sense to design one frontal and two posterior elements.

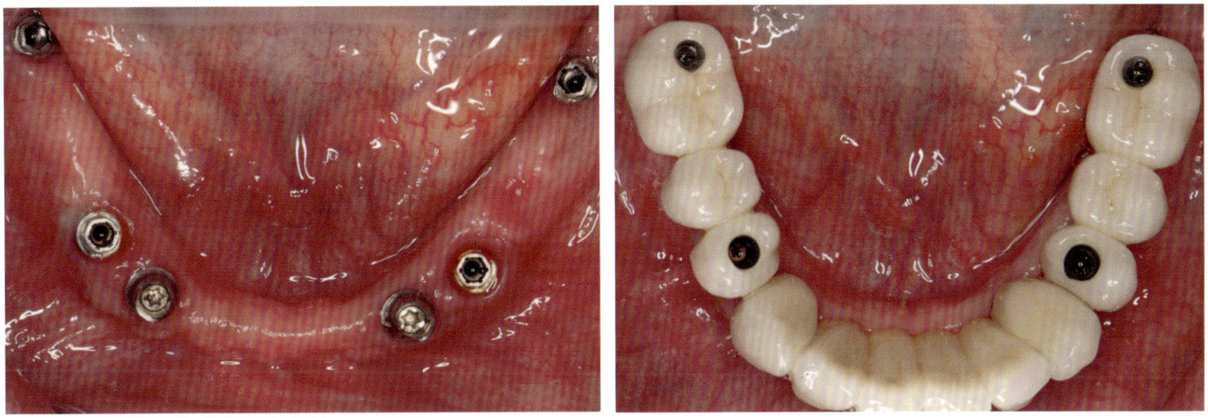

Figs. 117 a & b: Several bridge parts for a fixed restoration with implants in the posterior mandible

3.4.

Restoration of the edentulous maxilla

The quality of the bone in the maxilla is inferior to that in the mandible in most cases. Horizontal resorption is about twice as pronounced as vertical resorption in the anterior region [118], often resulting in very narrow alveolar ridges. Due to the often very thick mucosa, the bone situation is usually clinically inadequate. This may constitute a preoperative indication for three- dimensional imaging (CT/ DVT) [119].
As a rule, a minimum number of four implants is recommended for the implant-prosthetic restoration of the edentulous maxilla [120].
Before starting implant-prosthetic planning, special attention must be paid to the position of the smile line. The presence of a high smile line can be a decisive argument for the fabrication of a removable overdenture, which can well be superior in terms of function and esthetics. The lip profile can also be an indication for a removable denture if, for example, only a vestibular plastic shield can provide sufficient support for the labial soft tissue. Against this background, it is particularly important for restorations in the maxilla not to promise a fixed restoration too soon and to conduct a precise pre-implantological diagnosis and patient education in which the patient's expectations of the future dental prosthesis should be discussed as thoroughly as possible.
In the following, the treatment concepts 1-4 explain possible removable and fixed restoration options in the edentulous maxilla, ranging from a removable denture on four implants to extensive restoration using multiple implants and fixed crowns and bridges.

3.4.1.

Removable restorations in the edentulous maxilla

Treatment concept 1 (removable denture on four to five implants in the anterior maxilla)

To retain an implant-supported, mucosa-supported overdenture in the edentulous maxilla at least four implants should be inserted [121]. The denture is then designed as a coverdenture, whereby the palatal plate can be shortened in the posterior region and reduced palatally.

Bars with or without distal extensions, telescopic abutments, Locators or ballabutments can be used as mesostructures. (Figs. **118 – 120**). Due to the generally poorer bone quality in the maxilla, the author sees particular advantages in the primary splinting of the implants using a bar restoration. The flat design of the bar can also have advantages from a dental technology perspective when setting up and designing the front anterior teeth in the maxilla. In cases where the bone quality permits and good hygiene is a priority, planning secondary splinting using telescopic abutments also makes sense. When using Locators in a restoration, it should be noted that restoration can become problematic due to the atrophy-related typical "fanning out" of the implants, especially in the case of existing vestibular undercuts. With the exception of angled Locator systems, this procedure requires very parallel implant alignments so that the matrices can lock completely and effectively onto the male parts.

As mentioned at the beginning, retaining a removable, implant-supported and mucosa-supported overdenture is always possible if at least four implants of sufficient length can be placed.

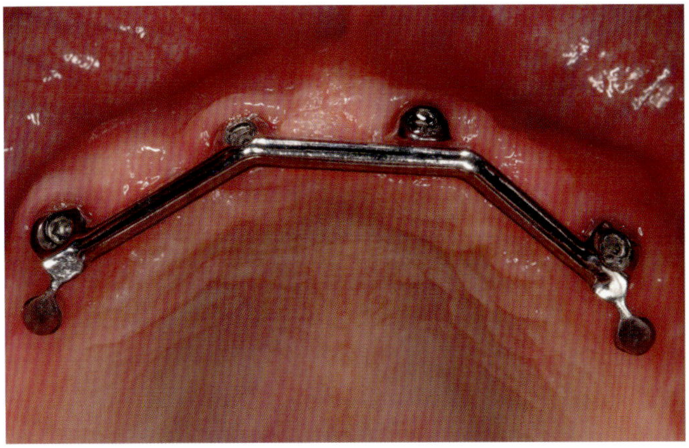

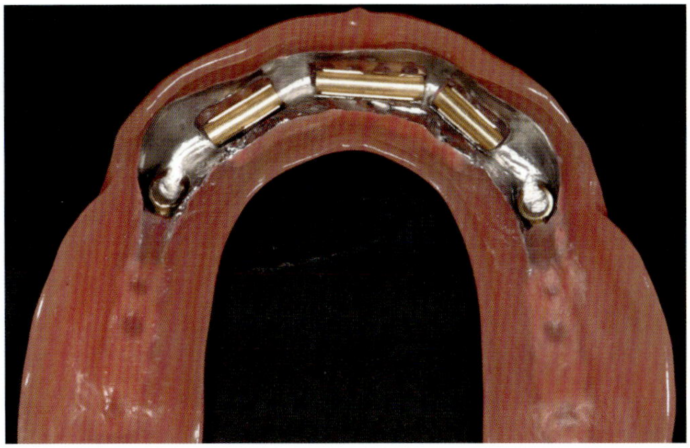

Figs. 118 a & b: Cast NPM bar on four implants in the edentulous maxilla with implant-supported, mucosa- supported denture

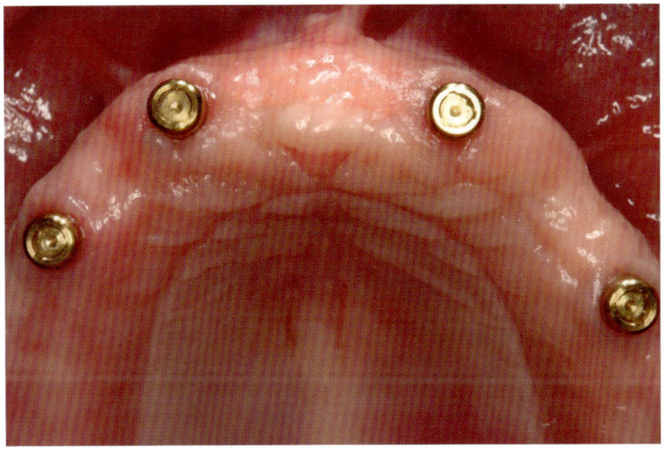

Fig. 119: Locators

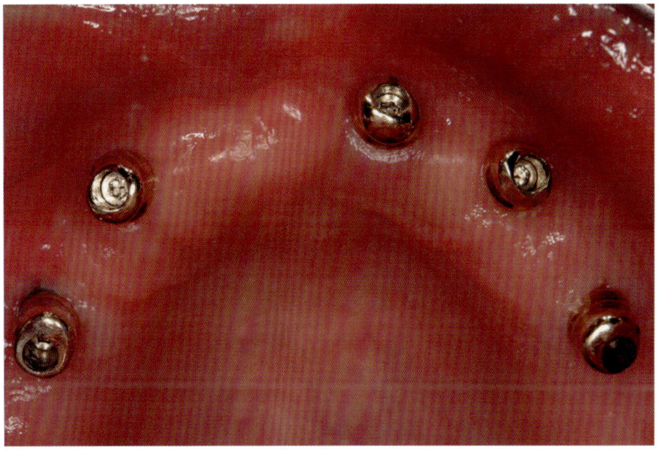

Fig. 120: Telescopic abutments

For this purpose, insertion of the distal implants at least into the canine, or even better into the premolar region, is a prerequisite for ensuring the most polygonal support possible. This may occasionally also require a sinus floor elevation in this treatment concept as a preparatory or simultaneous measure [122].

Similar to the design principles described, here too, the splinting of the implants should be made dependent on the bone quality, the primary stability, as well as the length and number of the implants, among other things. The expansion or the extent of the mucosa-borne prosthesis saddle is based on the extent of the implant support and can be reduced under certain circumstances depending on the extent of the support polygon.

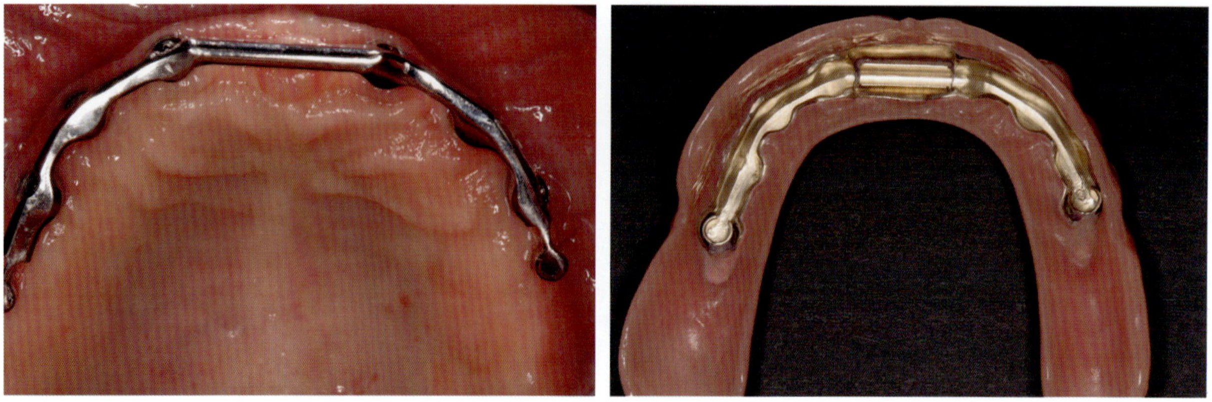

Figs. 121 a & b: Milled NPM bar on six implants and denture

Depending on the contour of the alveolar ridge, U- shaped or V-shaped, there are different design options for the bars in the maxilla, where the prefabricated components have increasingly been replaced by the milled components in recent years. Depending on the number and distribution of implants, the transition to treatment concept 2 can be seamless.

Treatment concept 2 (removable, implant- supported bar-retained overdenture or telescopic bridge on at least six implants)

A removable, implant-supported denture in the form of a telescopic bridge (Fig. **123**) or fully implant- supported bar-retained prosthesis (Figs. **121, 122, 124** and **125**) is possible on six or more implants [123].

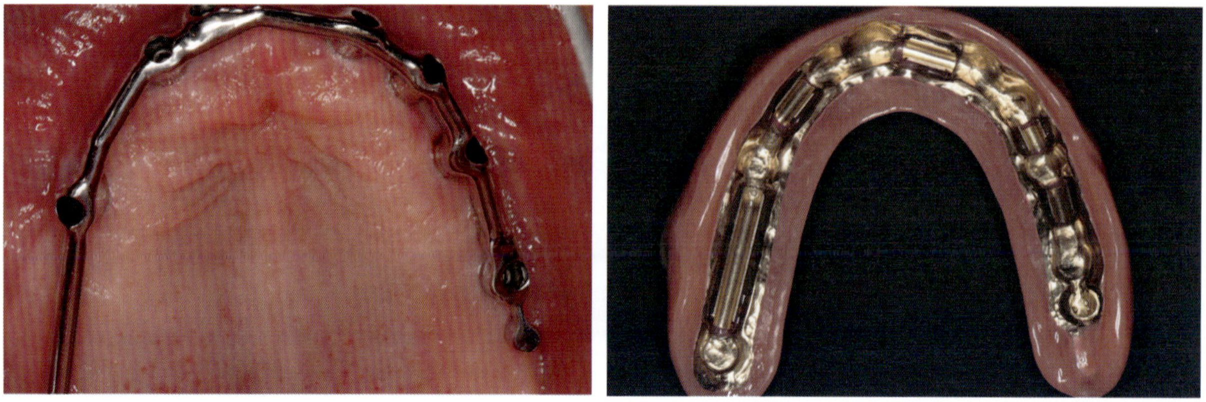

Figs. 122 a & b: Milled NPM bar on eight implants and a fully implant-supported denture

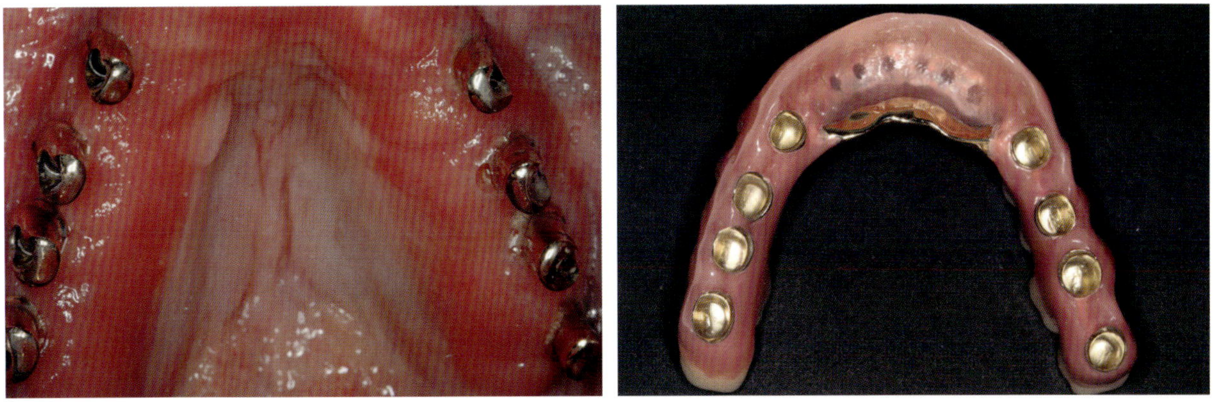

Figs. 123 a & b: Telescopic denture/bridge

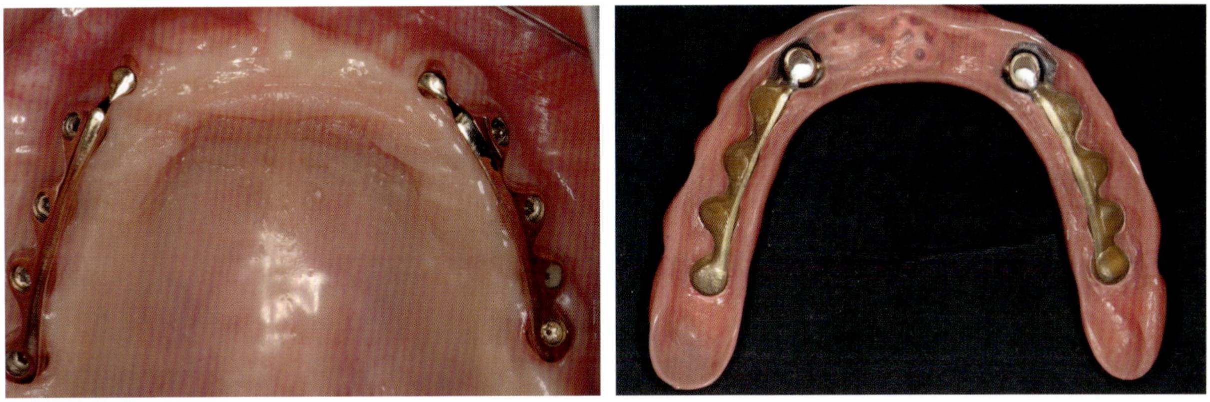

Figs. 124 a & b: Segmented cast gold bar and denture/bridge

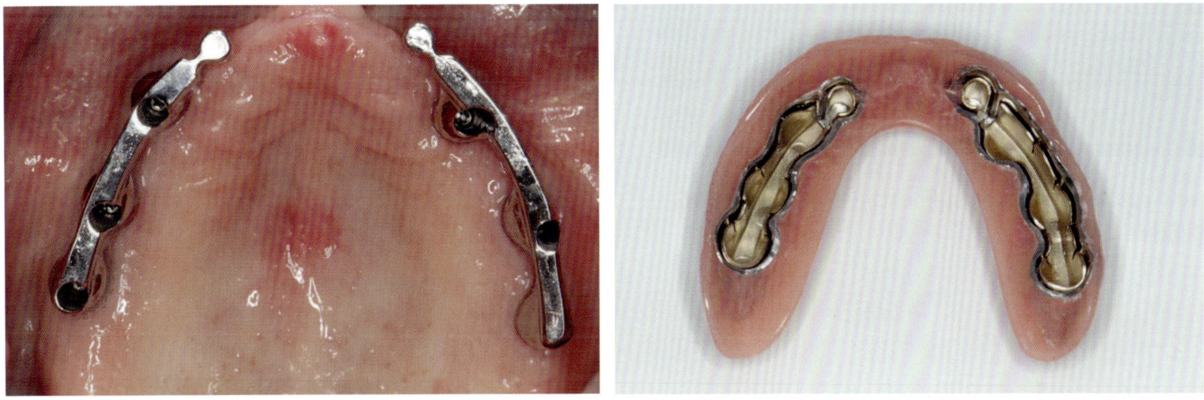

Figs. 125 a & b: Milled segmented bar and denture (Surgery/Iliac Crest Augmentation M. Erbe)

A denture supported by implants placed at sufficient distances from each other, even in the more posterior region, allows a significant reduction of the base and a more intricate, possibly bridge-like design. This concept is used in particular when the patient wishes to have a fixed restoration, but this is not feasible or advisable due to the limitations described above. The decisive factors include the patient's profile and smile line, as well as the interalveolar distance of the upper and lower jaw [124].
In the author's opinion, the decision as to whether comparable clinical situations should be restored with bars or telescopic crowns depends primarily on the factors bone quality and implant length. In such cases, it must be decided on an individual basis whether the advantage of primary splinting is considered essential

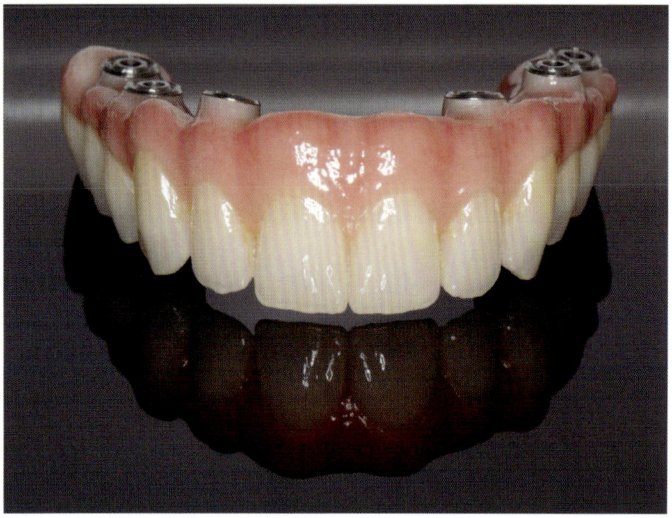

Fig. 126: Screw-retained implant-supported bridge made of zirconium oxide ceramic

3.4.2.

Fixed dentures in the edentulous maxilla

Treatment concept 3 (fixed, one-piece bridge or cantilever bridge on four to six implants)

Fixed, fully implant-supported dentures in the form of a one-piece screw-retained or cemented bridge are possible in the maxilla from a number of six, alternatively also on four to five implants [120, 125]. The prerequisite for treatment concept 3 is a favorable, preferably polygonal distribution of the abutments. If the implants are inserted more in the anterior part of the maxilla, the suprastructure can be designed as a shortened dental arch. In treatment concept 3, the set-up then extends to the premolar or first molar region. Here, the “All-on-4” treatment concept [126] offers an alternative with a reduced number of implants. The two anterior implants are inserted axially, the two posterior implants are inserted with distal angulation. However, this is a technique-sensitive procedure, that requires careful patient selection and thorough patient education [120]. The extensive, one-piece suprastructures made of metal-ceramic (see treatment concept on the following pages, Figs. **127 – 131**) or zirconium oxide ceramic (Fig. **126**), which are used in treatment concept 3, should preferably be designed screw-retained to reduce biological and technical complications [127].
Here, metal frameworks are to be given preference over ceramic frameworks. If the decision is made in favor of the ceramic version, it is advisable to design the parts subject to masticatory loads in particular, to be as monolithic as possible, to ensure low veneer thicknesses and freedom from tension, and to aim for perfect occlusion due to the high risk of “chipping” in veneered zirconium oxide frameworks.

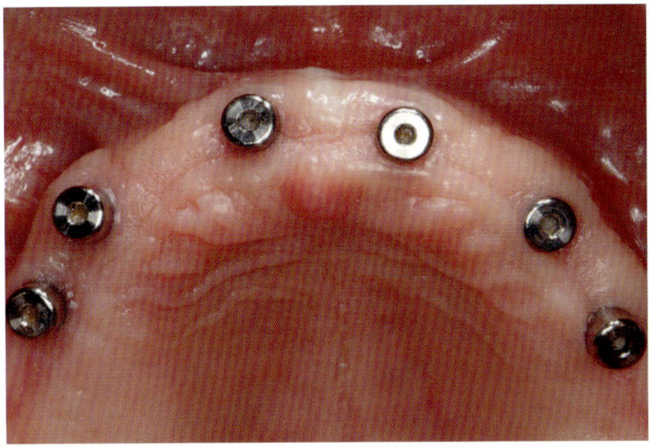

Fig. 127: Six implants in the edentulous maxilla

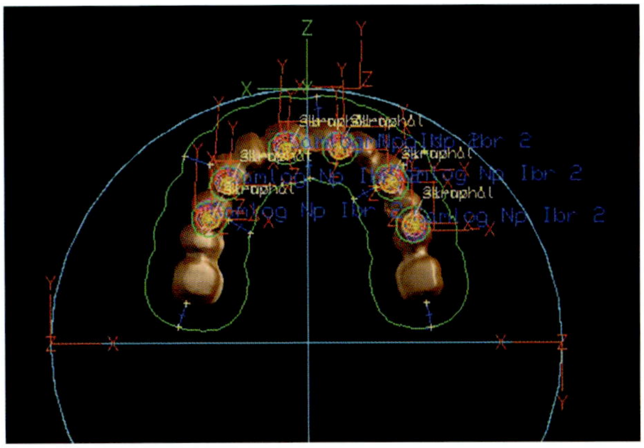

Fig. 128: Framework planning for CAD/CAM NPM framework

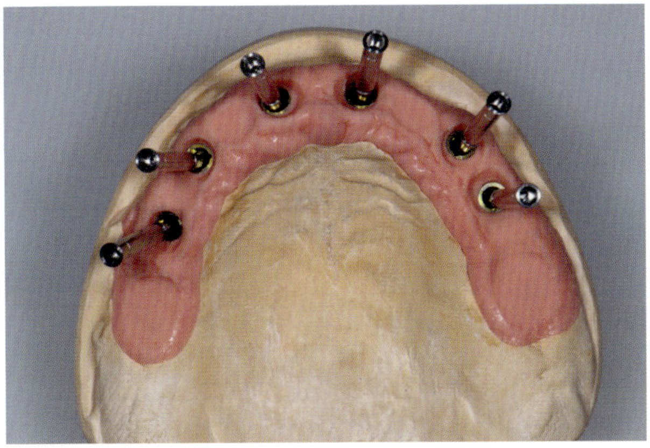

Fig. 129: Typically fan-shaped implant positions

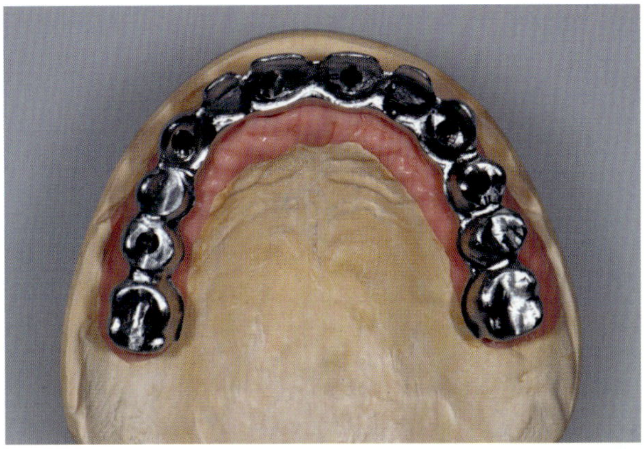

Fig.130: Screw access points placed in comfortable areas using angulated screw access holes

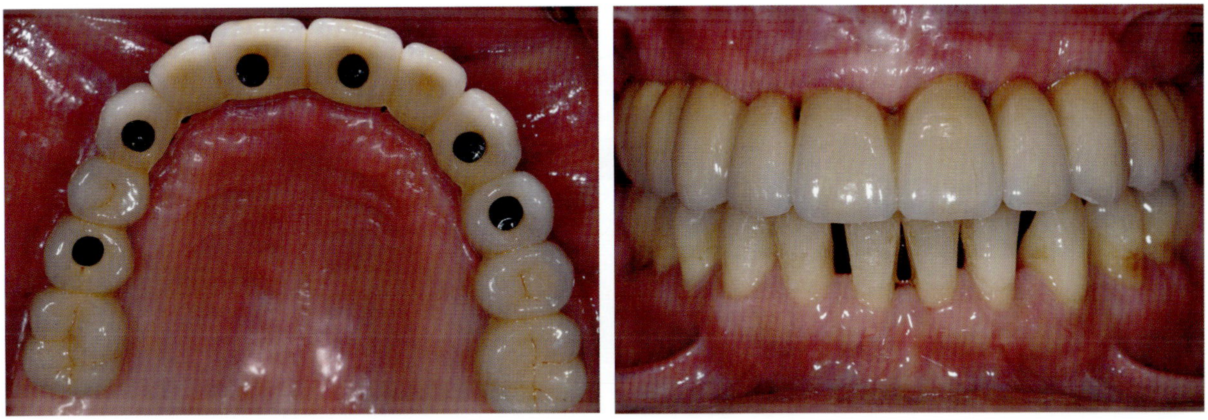

Figs. 131 a & b: Screw-retained metal-ceramic cantilever bridge

Treatment concept 4 (multi-unit fixed crown and bridge restoration with multiple implants – also in the posterior region – aiming at full-arch rehabilitation)

For extensive full-arch restoration up to the second molars (treatment concept 4), an insertion of at least eight implants is mandatory (Figs. **132 a & b**). As the anatomical prerequisites, especially in the posterior region, are rarely present from the outset for this type of restoration, alveolar ridge augmentation frequently has to be performed in the vertical dimension, but often also in the horizontal dimension. Interventions in the sense of soft tissue management may also prove necessary to achieve stable peri-implant soft tissue conditions.
Occasionally, as in treatment concept 3, pink ceramic material needs to be used to replace missing hard and soft tissue. As a matter of principle, it should be mentioned that in pronounced ridge atrophies, the desired fixed bridge restorations are usually more complicated from a dental technology point of view. Then, screw-retained mesostructures with cemented crowns may be necessary to bridge the interalveolar distance or to compensate for unfavorable implant positions. The option of angulated screw fixation represents an interesting addition to the range of therapies. These Restorations shown in Figures **133 a & b** have been largely replaced by this treatment option in the clinical practice of the author.

In particular, consistent planning is of great importance for treatment concepts 3 and 4, possibly also in the context of digital planning and workflow. Whereby the functional aspects should not be forgotten. The significantly higher masticatory loads on fully implant-supported restorations and the use of partially very hard materials must be taken into account in the interests of a precise and harmonious occlusion. The design of the occlusal surfaces should also take these factors into account and not be designed to be too "distinctive".

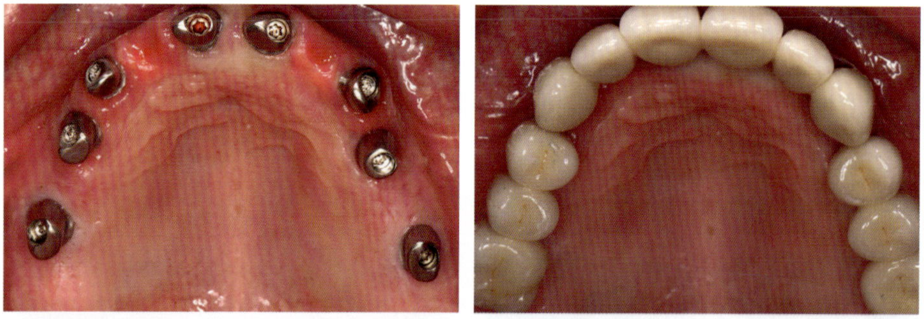

Figs. 132 a & b: Fixed cemented restoration (three bridge units) on eight implants

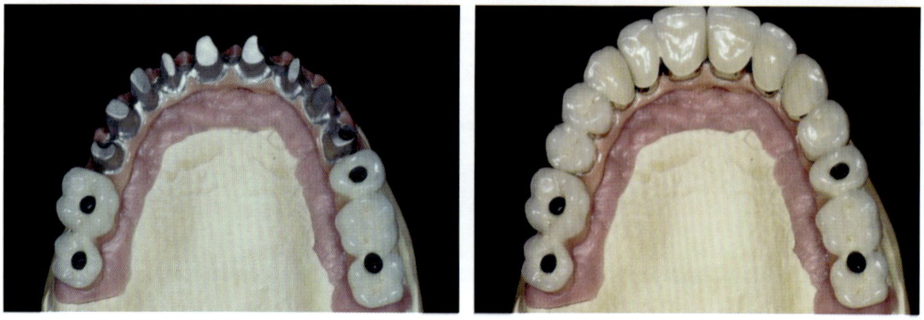

Figs. 133 a & b: Screw- retained mesostructure with anterior cemented crowns (image: H. Spiekermann)

Patient case: immediate restoration of the edentulous maxilla

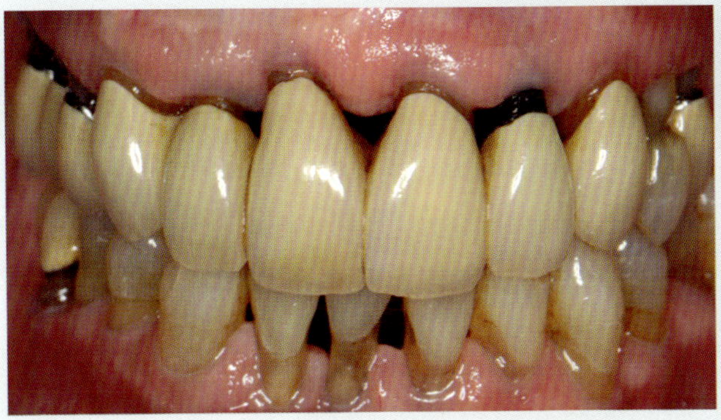

Fig. 134: The initial situation of a 64-year-old female patient

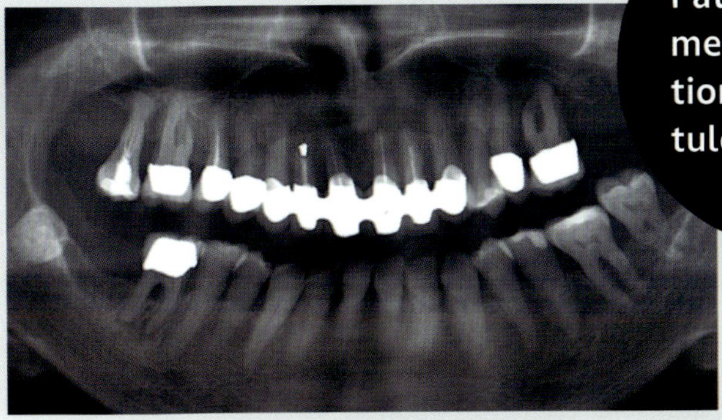

Fig. 135: The subsequent OPG shows the periodontally pre-damaged teeth

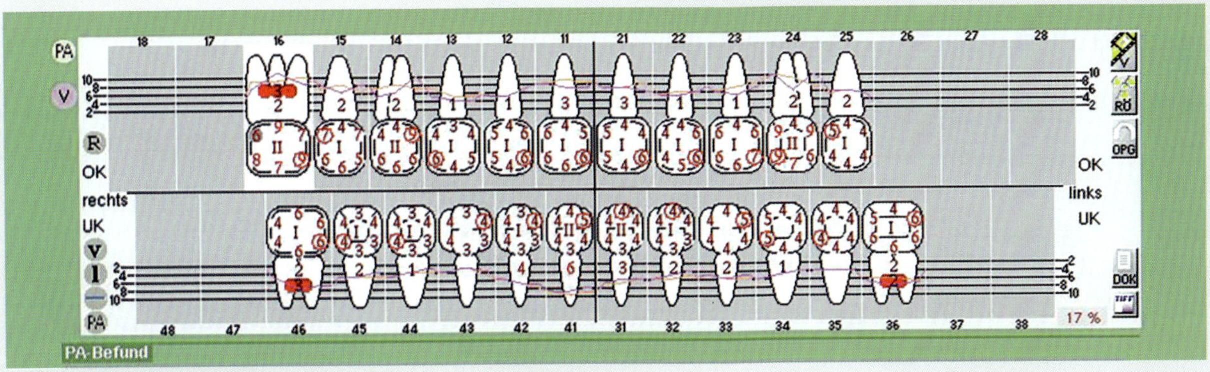

Fig. 136: Based on the probing depths during the re-evaluation according to FMD, a decision was made regarding the abutment prognosis in the maxilla and mandible, taking into account the patient's preference for a fixed and palate-free restoration.

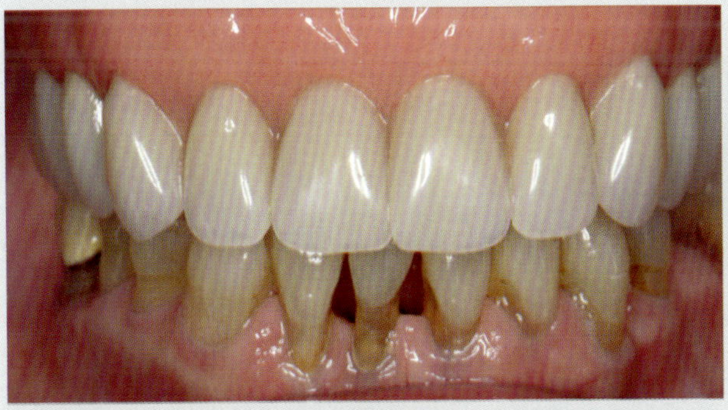

Fig. 137: Following extraction of the teeth that were not worth preserving, the immediate denture could be incorporated.

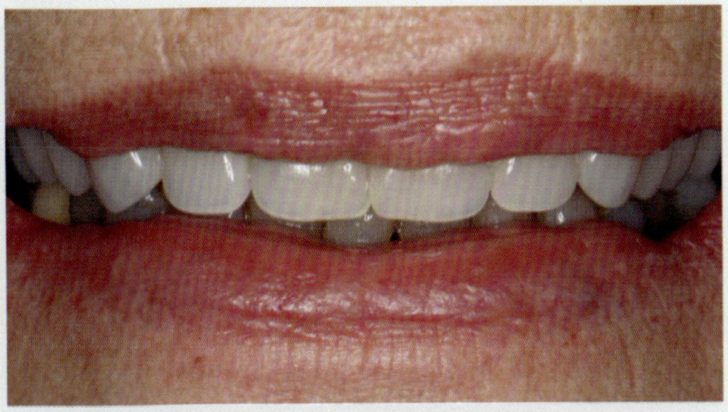

Fig. 138: The denture met the esthetic criteria in terms of tooth length, tooth positioning, and lip support.

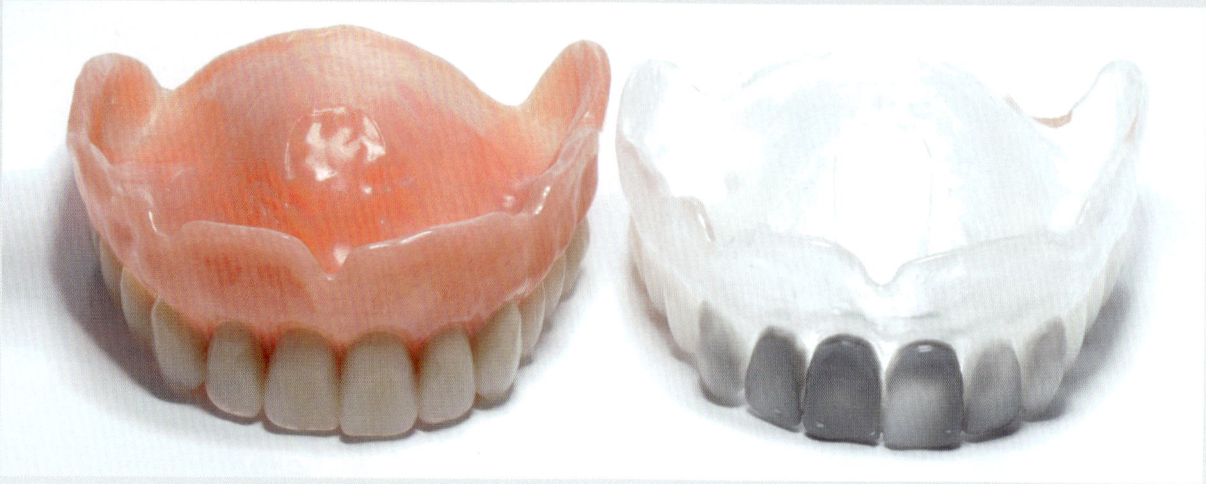

Fig. 139: The denture was duplicated for implant planning with DVT. The dental technician used barium sulfate containing teeth to visualize the tooth positions and fixed them to the glass-clear denture base.

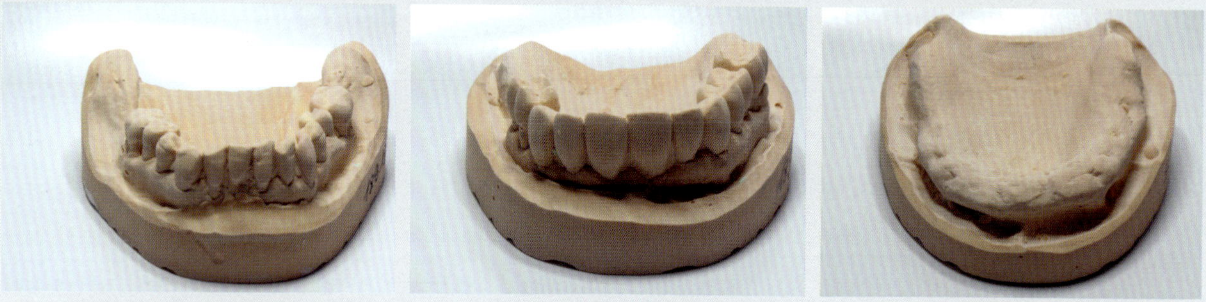

Figs. 140 a – c: Models for data matching and backward planning.

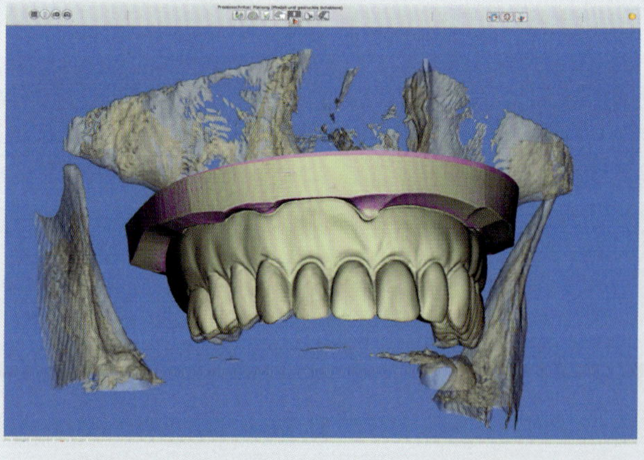

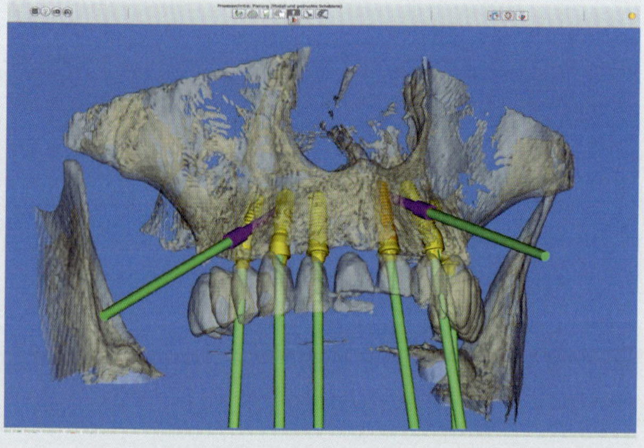

Fig. 141: The scanned setup and the data match from the DVT enabled optimal implant positioning I
Fig. 142: With the aid of the data sets stored in the library, the screw access channels and the position of the fixation screws were determined.

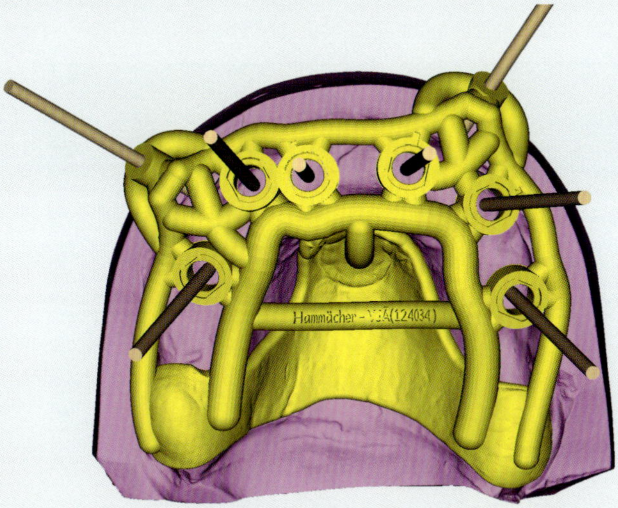

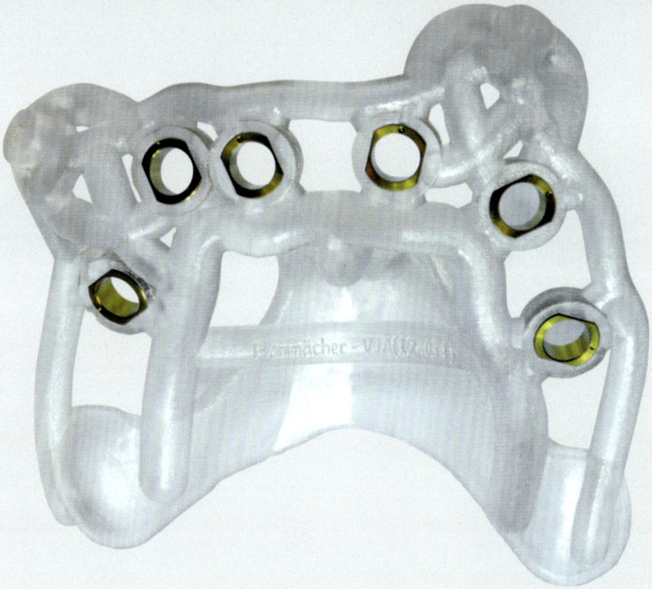

Fig. 143: The surgical guide was designed with recesses for the exact fixation of the guide sleeves as well as the anchor pins.

Fig. 144: The printed, skeletonized surgical guide provided an unobstructed view of the surgical area.

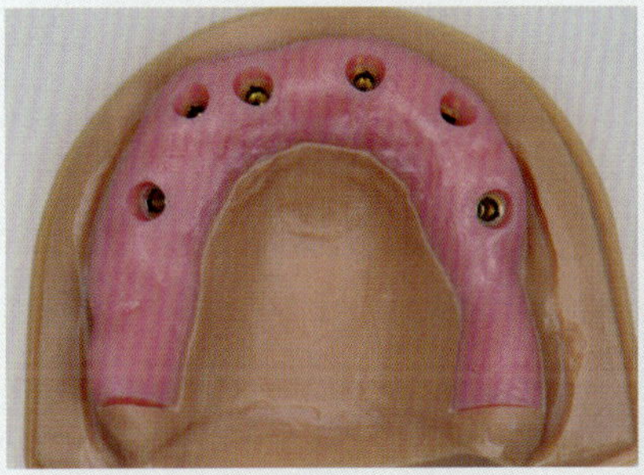

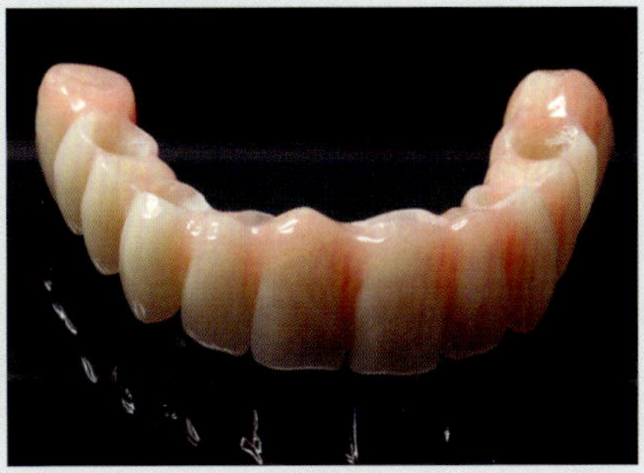

Fig. 145: Printed model with removable gingiva mask

Fig. 146: Preoperative provisional bridge, generously ground in the area of the titanium caps to be bonded.

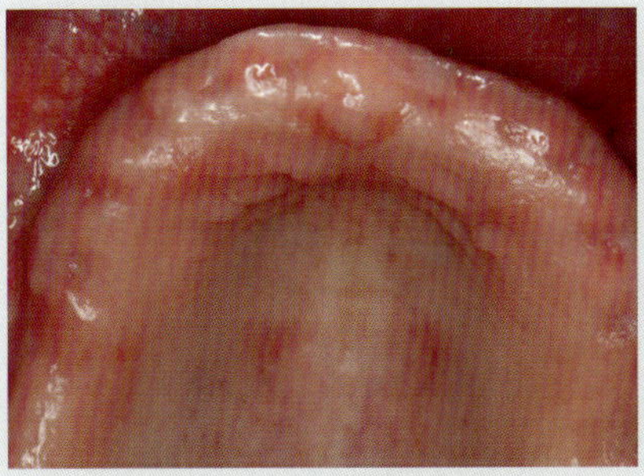

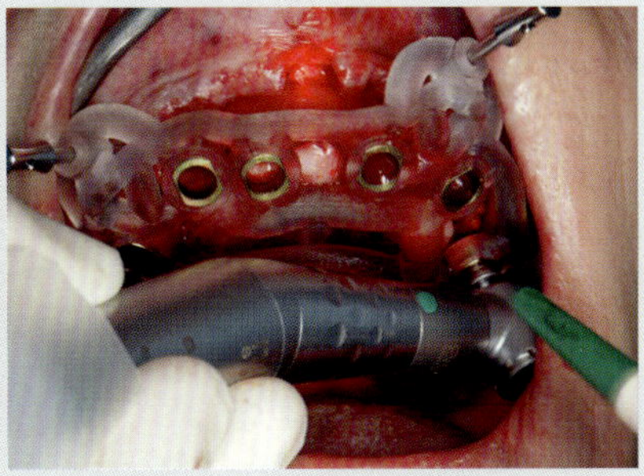

Fig. 147: The soft tissue in the maxilla had healed very well eight weeks after extraction of the teeth.

Fig. 148: The surgical guide was fixed to the bone after unfolding using two anchor pins.
(At that time, the planning software allowed fully guided drilling only for the initial osteotomy of the new implant system)

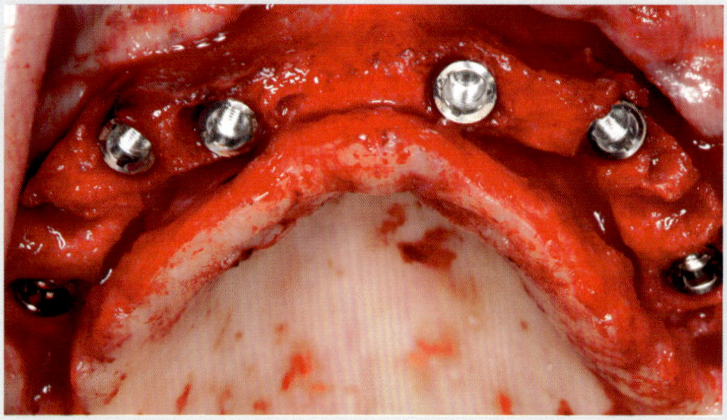

Fig. 149: Inserted implants

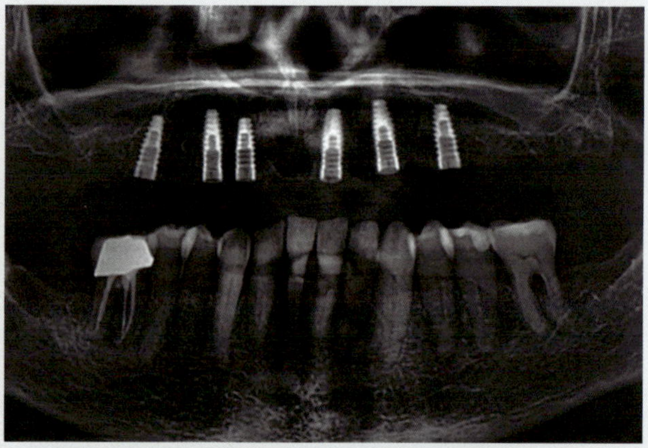

Fig. 150: Postoperative orthopantomogram

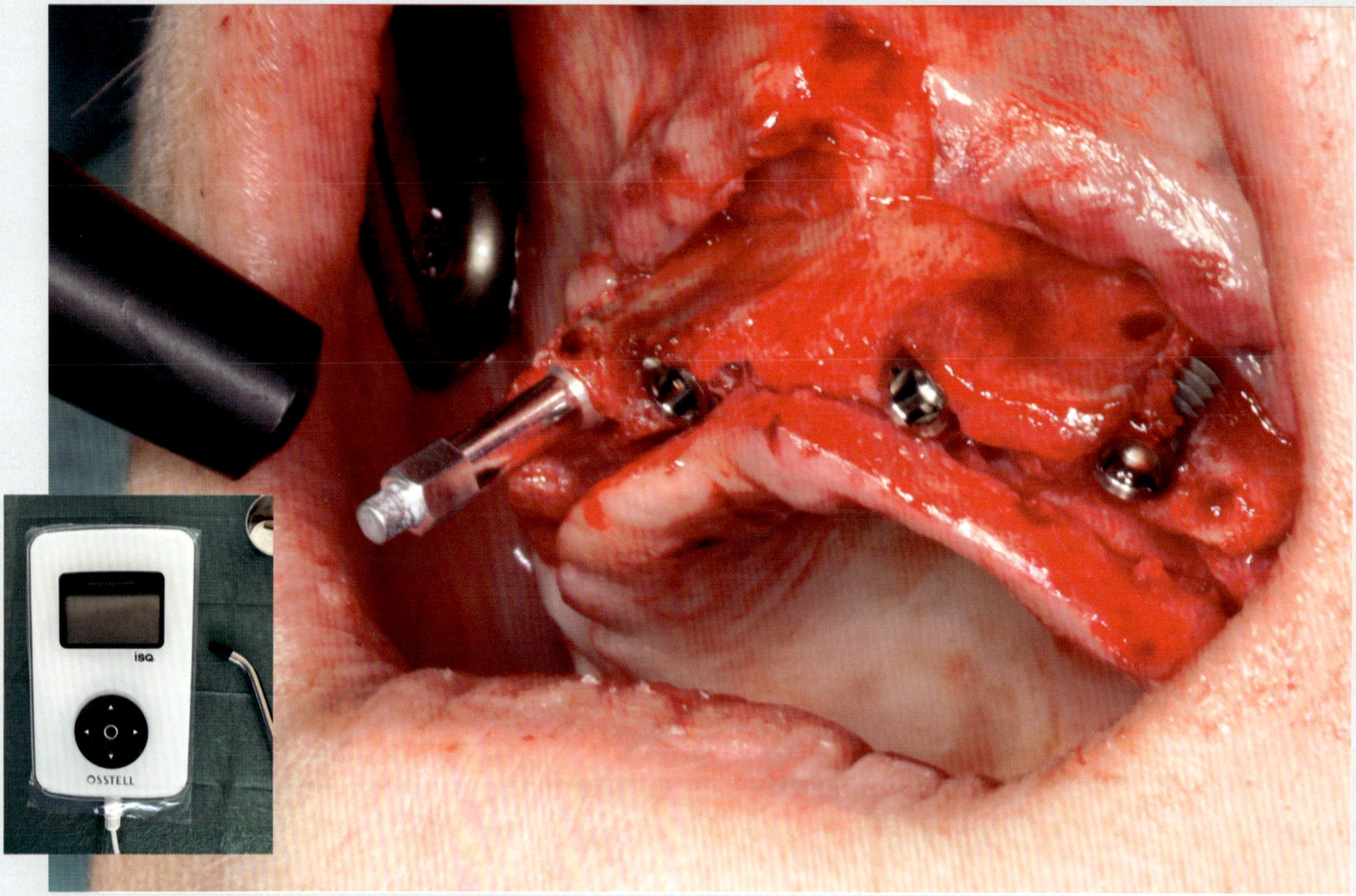

Figs. 151 a & b: The implants achieved high primary stability, measured using resonance frequency analysis (70–90 ISQ). The indication for immediate restoration was thus given.

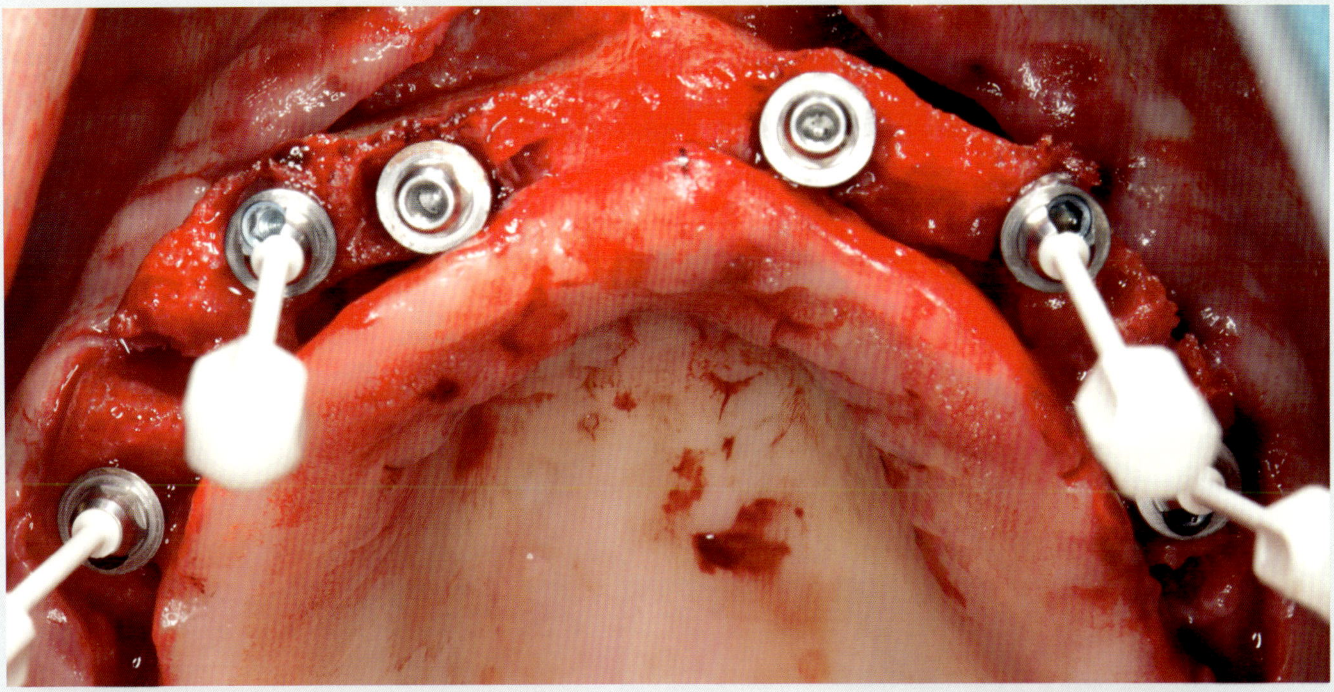

Fig. 152: The straight and angled bar abutments could be inserted safely using the flexible handle.

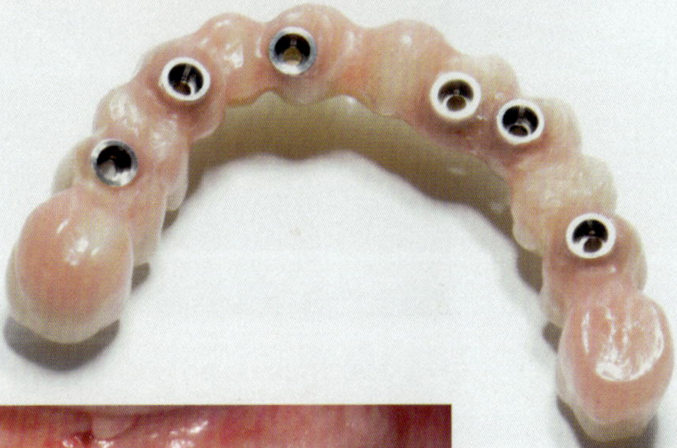

Fig. 153: After tension-free intraoral bonding of the titanium sleeves into the bridge, the basal portions were carefully finished and polished channels were created to achieve good oral hygiene.

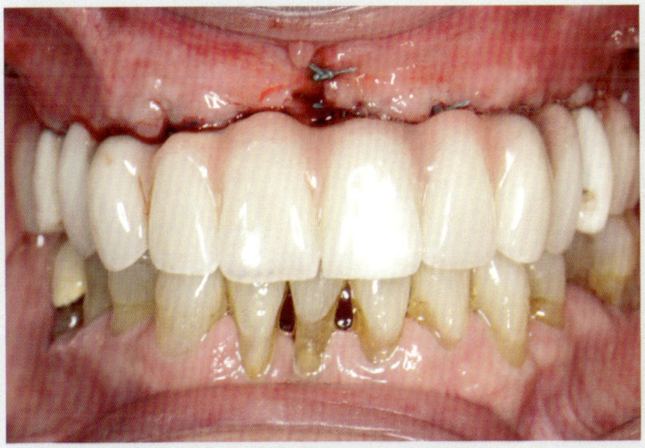

Fig. 154: The inserted provisional bridge immediately after surgical intervention

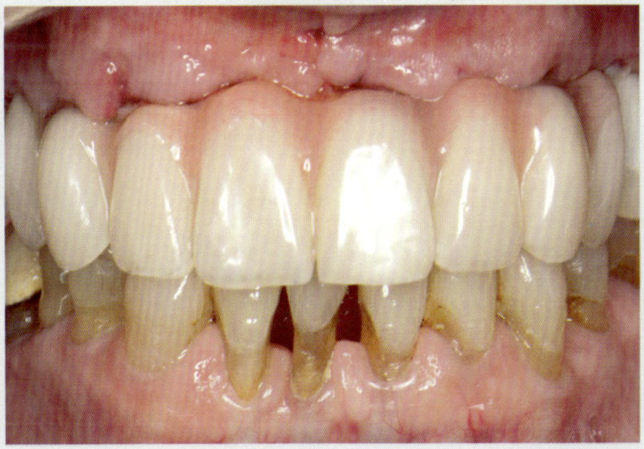

Fig. 155: The situation after suture removal ten days later

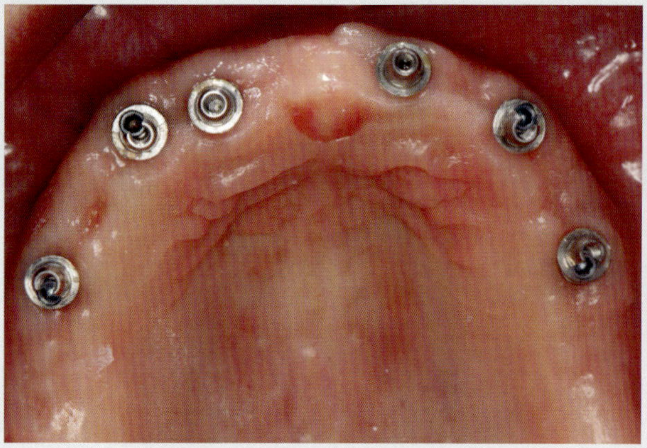

Fig. 156: Removal of the temporary restoration after five months of healing

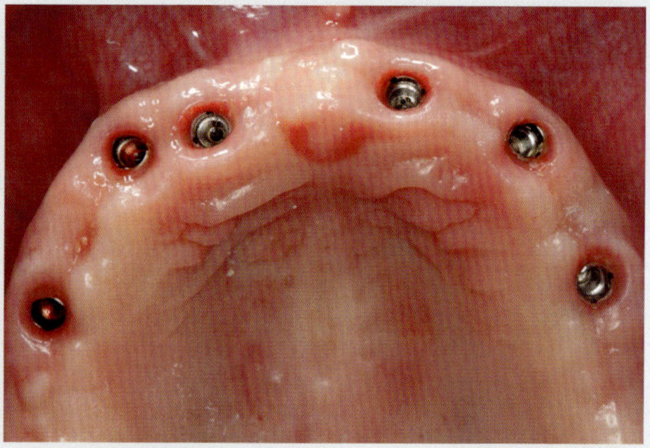

Fig. 157: The final restoration was performed from the implant shoulder.

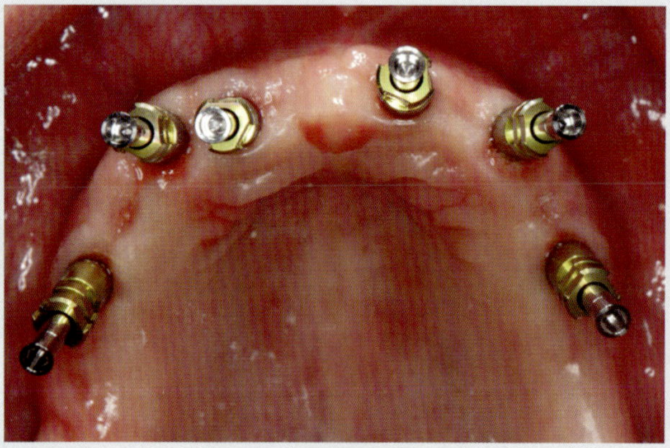

Fig. 158: Impression taking

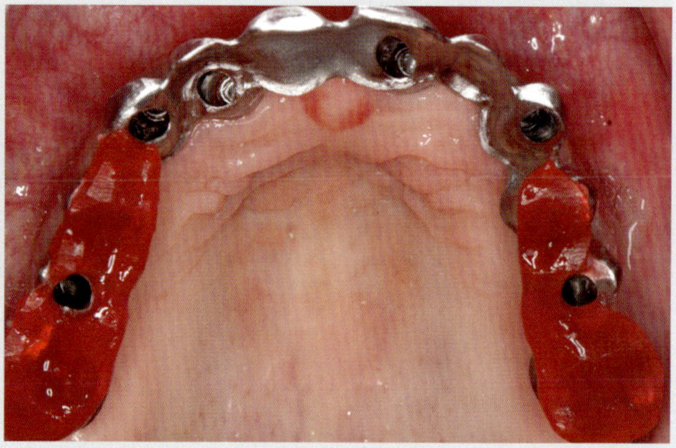

Fig. 159: Angled CAD/CAM non-precious metal framework screw-retained for try-in

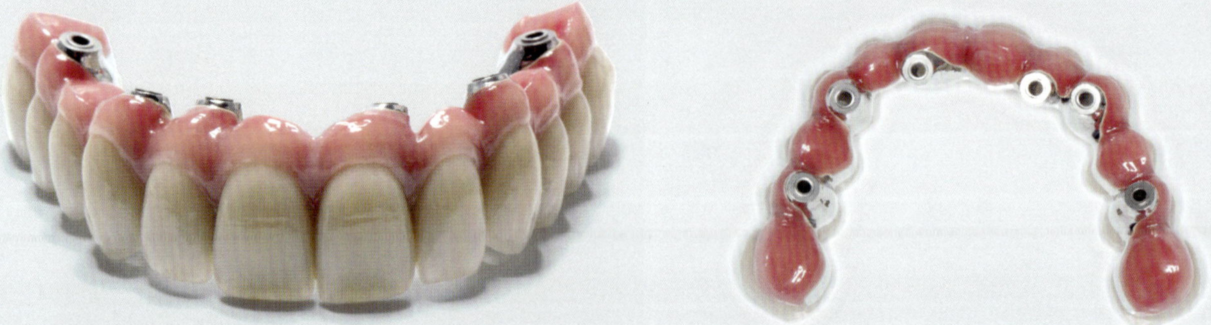

Figs. 160 a & b: Completed screw-retained metal-ceramic bridge with pink ceramic parts and convex basal design

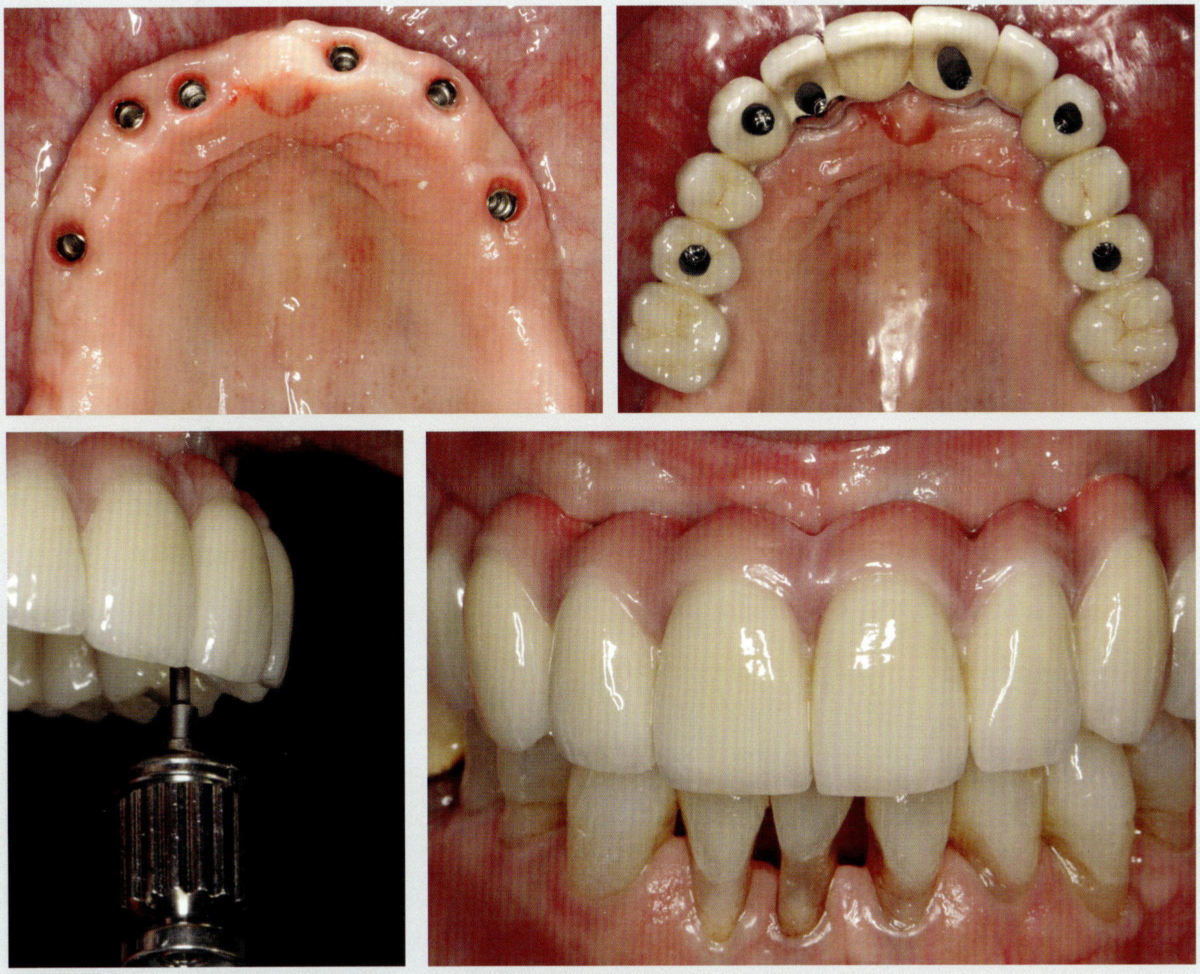

Figs. 161 a – d: Completed bridge screw-retained in the mouth

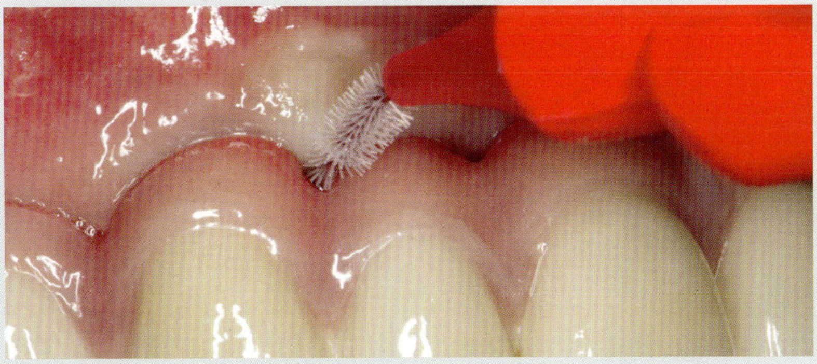

Fig. 162: Good cleanability owing to convex design and cleaning channels

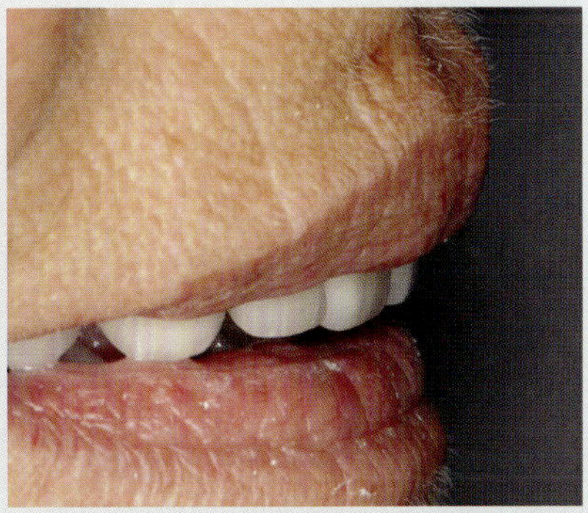

Fig. 163: Sufficient and appealing lip support

3.5.

Practical tips for preventing or managing complications

- Patients with an edentulous maxilla should never be promised a fixed restoration too soon. That is, unless consistent backward planning has been conducted, possibly whithin the digital workflow. But even then, early implant loss can jeopardize implementation of the planned restoration.
- When deciding on a fixed restoration for an edentulous maxilla, sufficient support of the perioral soft tissue must be given special consideration. Depending on the degree of atrophy and the skeletal positional relationship of the upper and lower jaw, it is not possible to achieve a fixed restoration in some cases, despite having a sufficient number of implants, without extremely extensive additional bone grafting.

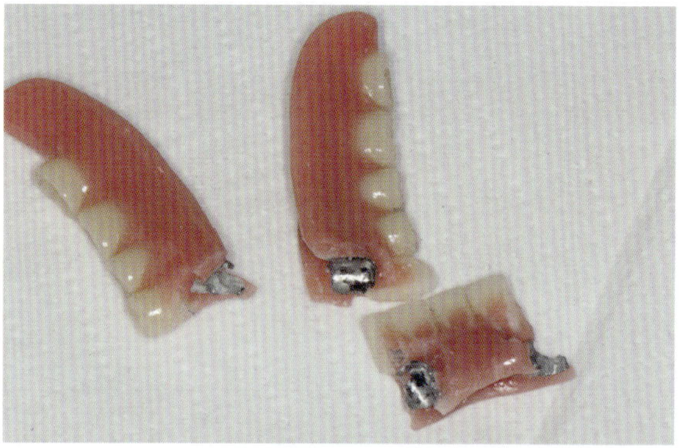

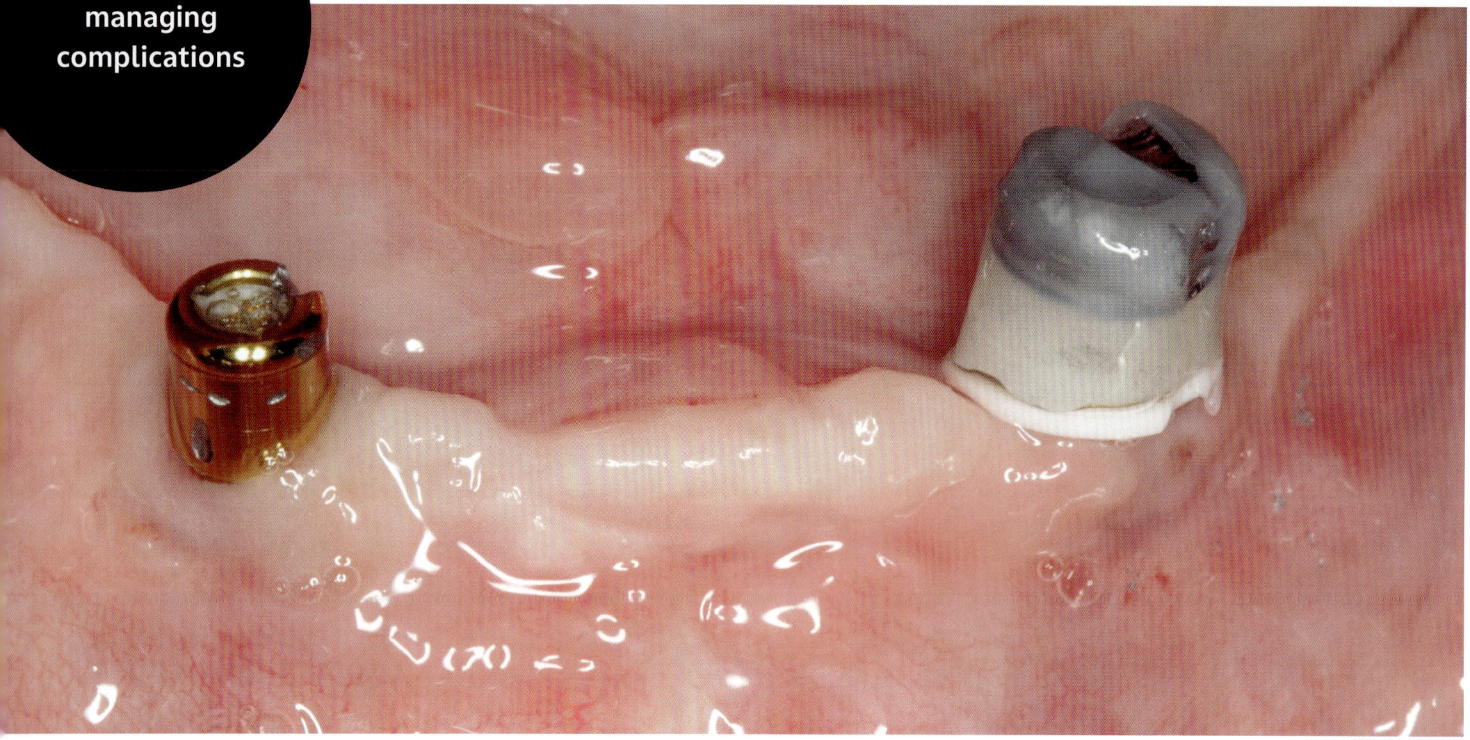

Figs. 164 a & b: Inadequate insulation and too much resin when bonding Locator matrices intraorally

- When planning the restoration with Locators, care should be taken to ensure that the implants are aligned in parallel. If they diverge too much, the rubber matrices resp. their metal sleeves wear out very quickly. Angled Locator systems may be the answer then.

- In the case of extensive restorations, whether fixed or removable, a wax-uo or esthetic try-in should always be performed before the framework is fabricated.

- In particular, with fixed metal-ceramic or all-ceramic restorations in edentulous patients, the significant increase in masticatory loads due to the missing receptors must be taken into account when the superstructure is in an absolutely rigid position. Perfect occlusion is then essential. In addition, a thin, soft splint should be fabricated for the patient.

- As a rule, the author recommends the insertion of four implants in the edentulous maxilla and two implants in the edentulous mandible as the minimum standard of restoration.

- When repairing or intraorally polymerizing bar or Locator matrices, ensure that the under-lying structures are adequately blocked out or isolated. (Figs. **164 a & b**).

- For a restoration with both milled bars as well as fixed bridge resorations, good hygienic capability must be ensured. Saddle-shaped supports should therefore be avoided.

- In the edentulous mandible, local keratinized gingiva should remain on the lingual side in particular when interforaminal implant exposure is performed. The movement there is greater than buccally, and free mucosal grafts to optimize the gingival conditions can be primarily integrated more predictably and successfully buccally.

3.6.

Conclusion

The use of implants to anchor removable dentures in the anterior edentulous maxilla and mandible usually leads to a significant improvement in the patient's quality of life. In the maxilla in particular, the possible reduction of the denture base depends on the number and distribution of the implants. The fan-shaped angulation of the implants often caused by the anatomy in the edentulous maxilla can make it difficult to provide a restoration with Locators. Fixed restorations in the maxilla and mandible with implants in the posterior regions often require extensive augmentation and complex surgical and prosthetic planning. Consistent backward planning, including three-dimensional X-ray diagnostics and virtual planning of implants and superstructures using digital workflow, can prove indispensable in such cases.
Fixed cantilever bridges, possibly also with angled distal implants, can be a treatment option. However, a reduction in the number of implants as well as immediate restoration for fixed restorations in the edentulous maxilla and mandible should be well considered and appropriate to the clinical and individual situation of the patient. Function, esthetics and long-term prognosis should be the guiding factors in treatment planning, along with the patient's wishes, age and medical history.

Further reading:

- Stefan Wolfart: Implant Prosthodontics A Patient-Oriented Strategy: Planning | Treatment Procedures | Longevity | Esthetics | Function | Dental Technology, 2016 Quintessence Publishing
- Happe A, Körner G: Erfolg mit Implantaten in der ästhetischen Zone: Parodontale, implantologische und restaurative Behandlungsstrategien, 2018. Berlin: Quintessenz Verlag
- Zuhr O, Hürzeler M: Plastic-Esthetic Periodontal and Implant Surgery A Microsurgical Approach 2012 Quintessence Publishing
- DGI e.Academy, the learning platform of the German Society for Implant Dentistry in collaboration with Springer publishers
- Beuer S, Stangl M: Der rote Faden: Dentalchirurgische Nahttechniken, 2019. teamwork media

Author for correspondence

Dr. Christian Hammächer
Dental Practice Center for Implant Dentistry, Periodontics and Prosthetics
Schumacherstraße 14
52062 Aachen

Conflict of interests

Christian Hammächer refers to the following relationships with manufacturers of products within the field of implant dentistry. Speaker fees received within the last five years: Camlog.

Literature

1. Müller HP, Eger T: Masticatory mucosa and periodontal phenotype: a review. Int J Periodontics Restorative Dent 2002; 22: 172–183
2. Linkevicius T, Apse P, Grybauskas S, Puisys A: The influence of soft tissue thickness on crestal bone changes around implants: a 1-year prospective controlled clinical trial. Int J Oral Maxillofac Implants 2009; 24: 712–719
3. Stein JM, Lintel-Höping N, Hammächer C, Kasaj A, Tamm M, Hanisch O: The gingival biotype: measurement of soft and hard tissue dimensions – a radiographic morphometric study. J Clin Periodontol 2013; 40: 1132–11
4. Tarnow D, Elian N, Fletcher P, Froum S, Magner A, Cho SC, Salama M, Salama H, Garber DA: Vertical distance from the crest of bone to the height of the interproximal papilla between adjacent implants. J Periodontol, 2003 Dec; 74 (12): 1785–1788
5. Jung RE, Schneider D, Ganeles J, Wismeijer D, Zwahlen M, Hämmerle CH, Tahmaseb A: Computer technology applications in surgical implant dentistry: a systematic review. Int J Oral Maxillofac Implants 2009; 24 Suppl: 92– 109
6. Schropp L, Wenzel A, Kostopoulos L, Karring T: Bone healing and soft tissue contour changes following single-tooth extraction: a clinical and radiographic 12-month prospective study. Int J Periodontics Restorative Dent
7. Wilson TG jr.: Guided tissue regeneration around dental implants in immediate and recent extraction sites: initial observations, Int J Periodontics Restorative Dent 1992; 12(3): 185–193
8. Novaes AB Jr, Vidigal Júnior GM, Novaes AB, Grisi MF, Polloni S, Rosa A: Immediate implants placed into infected sites: a histomorphometric study in dogs, Int J Oral Maxillofac Implants 1998 May–Jun; 13(3): 422–427
9. Chrcanovic BR, Martins MD, Wennerberg A: Immediate placement of implants into infected sites: a systematic review. Clin Implant Dent Relat Res 2015; 17 Suppl.: 1–16
10. Lee J, Park D, Koo KT, Seol YJ, Lee YM: Comparison of immediate implant-placement in infected and non-infected extraction-sockets: a systematic review and meta-analysis. Acta Odontol Scan 2018; 76(5): 338–345
11. Aráujo MG, Sukekava F, Wennström JL, Lindhe J: Ridge alterations following implant placement in fresh extraction sockets: an experimental study in the dog. J Clin Periodontol 2005; 32: 645–652
12. Blanco J, Nunez V, Aracil L, Munoz F, Ramos I: Ridge alterations following immediate implant placement in the dog: flap versus flapless surgery. J Clin Periodontol 2008 Jul; 35(7): 640–648
13. Grassi FR, Grassi R, Rapone B, Alemanno G, Balena A, Kalemaj Z: Dimensional changes of buccal bone plate in immediate implants inserted through open flap, open flap and bone grafting and flapless techniques: A randomized controlled clinical trial. Clin Oral Implants Res 2019; 30: 1155–1164
14. Chen ST, Darby IB, Reynolds EC, Clement JG: Immediate implant placement postextraction without flap elevation. J Periodontol 2009; 80: 163–172
15. Kan JY, Rungcharassaeng K, Lozada JL, Zimmerman G: Facial gingival tissue stability following immediate placement and provisionalization of maxillary anterior single implants: a 2-to-8-year follow-up. Int J Oral Maxillofac Implants 2011; 26: 179–187
16. Bäumer D, Zuhr O, Rebele S, Hürzeler M: Socket Shield Technique or immediate implant placement – clinical, radiographic and volumetric data after 5 years. Clin Oral Implants Res 2017; 28(11): 1450–1458
17. Wilson TG jr.: Guided tissue regeneration around dental implants in immediate and recent extraction sites: initial observations. Int J Periodontics Restorative Dent 1992; 12(3): 185–193
18. Botticelli D, Berglundh T, Lindhe J: Hard-tissue alterations following immediate implant placement in extraction sites. J Clin Periodontol 2004 Oct; 31(10): 820–828

19. Covani U, Cornelini R, Barone A: Bucco-lingual bone remodeling around implants placed into immediate extraction sockets: a case series. J Periodontol 2003 Feb; 74(2): 268–273
20. Fickl S, Zuhr O, Wachtel H, Kebschull M, Hürzeler MB: Hard tissue alterations after socket preservation with additional buccal overbuilding: a study in the beagle dog. J Clin Periodontol 2009 Oct; 36(10): 898–904
21. Aráujo MG, Lindhe J: Ridge preservation with the use of Bio-Oss collagen: A 6-month study in the dog. Clin Oral Implants Res 2009 May; 20(5): 433–440
22. Cardaropoli D, Tamagnone L. Roffredo A, Gaveglio L: Relationsship betwen the buccal plate thickness and the healing of postextraction sockets with/without ridge preservation. Int J Periodontics Restorative Dent. 2014; 34(2): 211–217
23. Spinato S, Galindo-Moreno P, Zaffe D, Bernardello F, Soardi CM: Is socket healing conditioned by buccal plate thickness? A clinical histologic study 4 months after mineralized human bone allografting. Clin Oral Impl Res 2014; 25(2): 120–126
24. Stimmelmayr M, Reichert T, Iglhaut G: Minimalinvasive Augmentationstechnik mittels Ridgepreservation und Socketseal in der ästhetisch anspruchsvollen Zone. Implantologie 2009; 17: 183–191
25. Stein JM, Hammächer C: Postextraction Socket Seal Surgery with an Epithelized Connective Tissue Graft using a Subpapillar Tunneling Procedure. Int J Periodontics Restorative Dent 2015; 35: 877–884
26. Azzi R, Etienne D: Recouvrement radiculaire et reconstruction papillaire par greffon conjonctif enfoui sous un lambeau vestibulaire tunnélisé et tracté coronairement. J Parodontol Implant Orale 1998; 17: 71–77
27. Zabalegui I, Sicilia A, Cambra J, Gil J, Sanz M: Treatment of multiple adjacent gingival recessions with the tunnel subepithelial connective tissue graft: a clinical report. Int J Periodontics Restorative Dent 1999; 19: 199– 206
28. Chen ST, Wilson TG Jr, Hämmerle C: Immediate or early placement of implants following tooth extraction: review of biologic basis, clinical procedures, and outcomes. Int J Oral Maxillofac Implants 2004; 19 Suppl: 12–25
29. Quirynen M, van Assche N, Botticelli D, Berglundh T: How does the timing of the implant placement to extraction affect outcome. Int J Oral Maxillofac Implants 2007; 22 Suppl: 203–223
30. Chen ST, Buser D: Esthetic outcomes following immediate an early implant placement in the anterior maxilla – a systematic review. Int J Oral Maxillofac Implants 2014; 29 Suppl: 186–215
31. Block MS, Mercante DE, Lirette D, Mohamed W, Ryser M, Castellon P: Prospective evaluation of immediate and delayed provisional single tooth restorations. J Oral Maxillofac Surg 2009 Nov; 67 (11 Suppl): 89–107
32. den Hartog L, Slater JJ, Vissink A, Meijyer HF, Raghoebar GM: Treatment outcome of immediate, early and conventional single-tooth-implants in the aesthetic zone: a systematic review to survival, bone level, soft-tissue, aesthetics and patient satisfaction. J Clin Periodontol 2008; 35(12): 1073–1086
33. Spear FM: Maintenance of the interdental papilla following anterior tooth removal. Pract Periodontics Aesthet Dent 1999 Jan–Feb; 11(1): 21–28.
34. Esposito M, Grusovin MG, Achille H, Coulthard P, Worthington HV: Interventions for replacing missing teeth: different times for loading dental implants. Cochrane Database Syst Rev 2009; Jan 21(1): CD003878
35. De Rouck T, Collys K, Cosyn J: Single-tooth replacement in the anterior maxilla by means of immediate implantation and provisionalization: a review. Int J Oral Maxillofac Implants 2008 Sep–Oct; 23(5): 897–904
36. Morton D, Jaffin R, Weber HP: Immediate restoration and loading of dental implants: clinical considerations and protocols. Int J Oral Maxillofac Implants 2004; vol. 19 Suppl: 103
37. Su H, Gonzalez-Martin O, Weisgold A, Lee E: Considerations of implant abutment and crown contour: critical contour and subcritical contour. Int J Periodontics Restorative Dent 2010; 30(4): 335–343
38. Katafuchi M, Weinstein BF, Leroux BG, Chen YW, Daubert DM: Restoration contour is a risk indicator for periimplantitis: A cross-sectional radiographic analysis. J Clin Periodontol 2018; 45(2): 225-232

39. Abrahamsson I, Berglundh T, Sekino S, Lindhe J: Tissue reactions to abutment shift: an experimental study in dogs. Clin Implant Dent Relat Res 2003; 5: 82–88
40. Wolfart S, Kern M: Optimierung der periimplantären Weichteilästhetik mit Provisorien. Implantologie 2008; 16: 171–182
41. Joda T, Wittneben JG, Bragger U: Digital implant impressions with the "Individualized Scanbody Technique" (IST) for emergence profile support. Clin Oral Impl Res 2013; 00: 1–3
42. Hammächer C, Weber V, Edelhoff D, Stein JM: Die „Doppelscan-Technik": Eine Methode zur digitalen Übertragung des Emergenzprofils. Implantologie 2013; 21(4): 385–404
43. Canullo L, Fedele GR, Ianello G, Jepsen S: Platform switching and marginal bone-level alterations: the result of a randomized-controlled trial. Clin Oral Implants Res 2010; 21: 115–121
44. Canullo L, Caneva M, Tallarico M: Ten year hard and soft tissue results of a pilot double blinded randomized controlled trial on immediately loaded postextractive implants using platform-switching concept. Clin Oral Implants Res 2017; 28: 1195–1203
45. Becker J, Ferrari D, Mihatovic I, Sahm N, Schaer A, Schwarz F: Stability of crestal bone level at platform-switched non-submerged titanium implants: a histomorphometrical study in dogs. J Clin Periodontol 2009; 36: 532–539
46. King GN, Hermann JS, Buser D, Cochran DL: Influence of the size of the microgap on crestal bone levels in non- submerged dental implants: a radiographic study in the canine mandible. J Periodontol 2002; 73: 1111–1117
47. Blum K, Wiest W. Fella C, Balles A, Dittmann J, Rack A, Maier D, Thomann R, Spies BC, Kohal RJ, Zabler S, Nelson K: Fatigue induced changes in conical implant-abutment connections. Dent Mater. 2015; 31(11): 1415– 1426
48. Schweiger J, Beuer F, Stimmelmayr M, Edelhoff D: CAD/CAM-generiert. Moderne Wege zum Implantatabutment. Zahnärztliche Mitteilungen 2012; 102: 2638–2646
49. Stimmelmayr M, Edelhoff D, Güth J, Erdelt K, Happe A, Beuer F: Wear of the titanium-titanium and the titanium- zirconia implant-abutment interface. A comparative in vitro study. Dent Mater 2012; 28: 1215–1224
50. Jung RE, Sailer I, Hämmerle CH, Attin T, Schmidlin P: In vitro color changes of soft tissues caused by restorative materials. Int J Periodontics Restorative Dent 2007; 27: 251–257
51. Fenner N, Hämmerle C, Sailer I, Jung RE: Long-term clinical, technical, and esthetic outcome of all-ceramic vs. titanium abutments on implant supporting single-tooth reconstructions alter at least 5 years. Clin Oral Implants Res 2016; 27: 716–723
52. Mitsias ME, Silva NR, Pines M, Stappert C, Thompson VP: Reliability and fatigue damage modes of zirconia and titanium abutments. Int J Prosthodont 2010; 23:56–59
53. Stimmelmayr M, Sagerer S, Erdelt K, Beuer F: In vitro fatigue and fracture strength testing of one-piece zirconia implant abutments an zirconia implant abutments connected to titanium cores. Int J Oral Maxillofac Implants 2013; 28(2): 488–493
54. Amorfini L, Storelli S, Mosca D, Scanferla M, Romeo E: Comparison of cemented vs screw-retained, customized computer-aieded design/computer assisted manufacture zirconia abutments für esthetically located single-tooth- implants: A 10 – year randomized prospective study. Int J Prosthodont 2018; 31: 359–36
55. Zetu L, Wang HL: Management of inter -dental/inter-implant papilla. J Clin Periodontol 2005; 32: 831–839
56. Nickenig HJ, Schäfer C, Spiekermann H: Survival and complication rates of combined tooth-implant-supported fixed partial dentures. Clin Oral Implants Res 2006; 17: 506–511
57. Burkhardt R, Joss A, Lang NP: Soft tissue dehiscence coverage around endosseous implants: a prospective cohort study. Clin Oral Implants Res 2008; 19: 451–457

58. Roccuzzo M, Gaudioso L, Bunino M, Dalmasso P: Surgical treatment of buccal soft tissue recessions around single implants: 1-year results from a prospective pilot study. Clin Oral Impl Res 2014; 25: 641–646
59. Zucchelli G, Mazzotti C, Mounssif I, Mele M, Stefanini M, Montebugnoli L: A novel surgical-prosthetic approach for soft tissue dehiscence coverage around single implant. Clin Oral Implant Res 2013; 24: 957–962
60. Cairo F, Barbato L, Selvaggi F, Baielli MG, Piattelli A, Chambrone L: Surgical procedures for soft tissue augmentation at implant sites. A systematic review and meta-analysis of randomized controlled trials. Clin Implant Dent Relat Res 2019; 21: 1262–1270
61. Nickenig HJ, Spiekermann H: CT/DVT-basierte implantatprothetische Führungsschablonen vs. traditionelle Orientierungsschablone. Z Zahnärztliche Impl 2006; 22: 272–280
62. Vercruyssen M, Hultin M, Van Assche N, Svensson K, Naert I, Quirynen M: Guided surgery: accuracy and efficacy. Periodontol 2000, 2014; 66(1): 228–246
63. Consensus report – reconstructions on implants. The third EAO Consensus Conference 2012. Heydecke G, Zwahlen M, Nico A, Nisan D, Payer M, Renouard F, Grohmann P, Mühlemann S. Joda T: What is the optimal number of implants for fixed reconstructions: a systematic review. Clin Oral Implants Res 2012; 23 (Suppl.6): 217–228
64. Stoumpis C, Kohal RJ: To splint or not to splint oral implants in the implant-supported overdenture therapy? A systematic literature review. J Oral Rehabil 2011; 38 (11): 857–869
65. Ravidà A, Tattan M, Askar H, Barootchi S, Tavelli L, Wang HL: Comparison of three different types of implant- supported fixed dental prostheses: A long-term retrospective study of clinical outcomes and cost – effectiveness. Clin Oral Implants res 2019; 30: 295–305
66. Fransson C, Wennsgtröm J, Tomasi C, Berglundh T: Extent of peri-implantitis-associated bone loss. J Clin Periodontol. 2009; 36(4): 357–363
67. Meijer HJA, Boven C, Delli K, Raghoebar GM: Is there an effect of crown-to-implant ratio on implant treatment outcomes? A systematic review. Clin Oral Implants Res 2018; 29 (Suppl 18): 243–252
68. Steinebrunner L, Wolfart S, Ludwig K, Kern M: Implant-abutment interface design affects fatigue and fracture strength of implants. Clin Oral Implants 2008 Res 19(12): 1276–1284
69. Strub JR, Gerds T: Fracture strength and failure mode of five different single-tooth implant-abutment combinations. Int J Prothodont 2003; 16(2): 167–171
70. Guichet DL, Caputo AA, Choi H, Sorensen JA: Passivity of fit and marginal opening in screw-or cement-retained implant fixed partial denture designs. Int J Oral Maxillofac Implants 2000 Mar–Apr; 15 (2): 239–246
71. Jung RE, Pjetursson BE, Glauser R, Zembic A, Zwahlen M, Lang NP: A systematic review of the 5-year survival and complication rates of implant-supported single crowns. Clin Oral Implants Res, 2008 Feb, 19(2): 119–30
72. Korsch M, Obst U, Walther W: Cement-associated peri-implantitis: a retrospective clinical oberservational study of fixed implant-supported restorations unsing a methacrylate cement. Clin Oral Implants Res 2013 April 21
73. Rosa L, Borba M, Mallmann F, Fornari F, Della Bona A: Influences of screw access hole and mechanical cycling on the fracture load of implant-supported crowns. Int J Prosthodont 2019; 32: 423–429
74. Sailer I. Mühlemann S, Zwahlen M, Hämmerle CHF, Schneider D: Cemented and screw-retained implant reconstructions: A systematic review of the survival and complication rates. Clin Oral Impl Res 2012; 23: 163– 201
75. Salvi G., Brägger U: Mechanical and technical risks in implant therapy. Int J Oral Maxillofac Implants 2009; 24: 69–85
76. Wittneben JG, Millen C, Brägger U: Clinical performance of screw-versus cement retained fixed implant- supported reconstructions: a systematic review. Int J Oral Maxillfac Implants 2014; 29 (Suppl): 84–98

77. Stimmelmayr M, Edelhoff D, Güth J, Erdelt K, Happe A, Beuer F: Wear of the titanium-titanium and the titanium- zirconia implant-abutment interface. A comparative in vitro study. Dent Mater 2012; 28: 1215–1224
78. Pitta J, Hicklin SP, Fehmer V, Boldt J, Gierthmuehlen PC, Sailer I: Mechanical stability of zirconia meso-abutmments bonded to titanium bases restored with diffent momolithic all-ceramic crowns. Int J Oral Maxillofac Im plants 2019; 34: 1091–1097
79. Nouh I, Kern M, Sabet AE, Aboelfadi AK, Hamdy AM, Chaar MS: Mechanical behaviour of posterior all-ceramic hybrid-abutment-crowns versus hybrid-abutments with separate crowns-a laboratory-study. Clin Oral Implants res 2019; 30: 90–98
80. Mitsias ME, Silva NR, Pines M, Stappert C, Thompson VP: Reliability and fatigue damage modes of zirconia and titanium abutments. Int J Prosthodont 2010; 23: 56–59
81. Friberg B, Ahmadzai M: A prospective study on single tooth reconstructions using parallel walled implants with internal connection (Nobel Parallel CC) and abutments with angulated screw channels (ASC). Clin Implant Dent Relat Res 2009; 21: 226–231
82. Pjetursson BE, Brägger U, Lang NP, Zwahlen M: Comparison of survival and complication rates of tooth-supported fixed dental prostheses (FDPs) and implant-supported FDPs and single crowns (Scs), Clin Oral Implants Res, 2007 Jun, 18 Suppl 3: 97–113
83. Lang NP, Pjetursson BE, Tan K, Brägger U, Egger M, Zwahlen M: A systematic review of the survival and complication rates of fixed partial dentures (FPDs) after an observation period of at least 5 years. II. Combined tooth-implant-supported FPDs. Clin Oral Impl Res 2005; 15(6): 643–653
84. Olsson M, Gunne J, Astrand P, Borg K: Bridges supported by free-standing implants versus bridges supported by tooth and implant: A five-year prospective study. Clin Oral Implants 1990; Res 6: 137–144
85. Gunne J, Astrand P, Lindh T, Borg K, Olsson M: Tooth-implant and implant supported fixed partial dentures: a 10-year report. Int J Prosthodont 1999 May–Jun; 12(3): 216–21
86. Nickenig HJ, Schäfer C, Spiekermann H: Survival and complication rates of combined tooth-implant-supported fixed partial dentures, Clin Oral Implants Res 2006 Oct; 17(5): 506–11
87. Weber HP, Zimerina Y: Survival and complication rates of fixed partial dentures supported by a combination of teeth and implants. J Evid Based Dent Pract. 2012
88. Richter, EJ (Med.-Habil Aachen 1992): Kaukraftmessungen in vivo mittels Kraftmesszellen in den Implantataufbauteilen von IMZ-Implantaten
89. Spiekermann H: Farbatlanten der Zahnmedizin Bd. 10, Implantologie, Hrsg. K.H. Rateitschak und H. F. Wolf, Thieme Verlag 1994
90. Heinemann F, Mundt T, Böttger S, Biffar R: Die Greifswalder Verbundbrücke aus Zirkonoxid. Quintessenz 2005; 56(11): 1183–90
91. Hammächer C, Yildirim M, Hanisch O, Spiekermann H: Strategische Pfeilerimplantate zur Abstützung von herausnehmbaren Teilprothese oder teleskopierenden Brücken, in: Quintessenz 53, 2002: 603–611
92. Fobbe H, Rammelsberg P, Lorenzo Bermejo J, Kappel S: The up- to-11-year survival and success of implants and abutments teeth under solely implant-supported and combined tooth-implant-supported double crown- retained removable dentures. Clin Oral Implants Res 2019; 30: 1134–1141
93. Krennmair G, Krainhöfner M, Waldenberger O, Piehslinger E: Dental implants as strategic supplementary abutments for implant-tooth-supported telescopic crown-retained maxillary dentures: a retrospective follow-up- study to 9 years. Int J Prosthodont 2007; 20(6): 617–622
94. Kern JS, Hanisch O, Hammächer C, Yildirim M, Wolfart S: Telescopic crowns on implants and teeth: evaluation of a clinical study after 8 to 12 years. Int J Oral Maxillofac Implants 2019; 34: 977–986

95. Semper-Hoff W, Kraft S, Stíller S, Mehrhof J, Nelson K: Analytical and experimental position stability of the abutment in different dental implant systems with a conical implant-abutment connection. Clin Oral Investig. 2013 Apr; 17(3): 1017–1023
96. Babbush CA: Provisional implants: surgical and prosthetic aspects. Implant Dent, 2001, 10(2): 113–120
97. Mombelli A, Marxer M, Gaberthüel T, Grunder U, Lang NP: The microbiota of osseointegrated implants in patients with a history of periodontal disease. J Clin Periodontol, 1995 Feb, 22(2): 124–130
98. Sumida S, Ishihara K, Kishi M, Okuda K: Transmission of periodontal disease-associated bacteria from teeth to osseointegrated implant regions. Int J Oral Maxillofac Implants, 2002 Sep-Oct, 17(5): 696–702
99. Lekholm U, Zarb GA: Patient selection and preparation, in: Brånemark PI, Zarb GA, Albrektsson T: Tissue- integrated prosthesis, osseointegration in clinical dentistry, Quintessenz Berlin, 1985
100. Spiekermann H et al.: Farbatlanten der Zahnmedizin Bd. 10, Implantologie, Hrsg. Klaus H. Rateitschak und Herbert F. Wolf, Thieme Verlag Stuttgart, 1994
101. Malo P, de Araujo Nobre M, Lopes A, Francischone C, Rigolizzo M: „All-on-four" immediate function concept für completely edentulous maxillae: a clincial report on the medium (3 years) and long-term (5 years) outcomes. Clin Implant Dent Relat. Res. 2012; 14 Suppl.1: e139–e150
102. Pozzi A, Holst S, Fabbri G, Tallarico M: Clinical reliability of CAD/CAM cross-arch zirconia bridges on immediately loaded implants placed with computer assisted/template-guided surgery: a retrospective study with a follow-up between 3 and 5 years. Clin Implant Dent Relat Res 2015; 17 (Suppl 1): e86–96
103. Meloni SM, Tallarico M, Pisano M, Xhanari E, Canullo L: Immediate loading of fixed complete denture prostheses supported by 4–8 implants placed using guided surgery: A 5-year prospective study on 66 patients with 356 implants. Clin Implant Dent Relat Res 2017
104. Heydecke G, Boudrias P, Awad MA, De Albuquerque RF, Lund JP, Feine JS: Within-subject comparison of maxillary fixed removable implant prostheses: Patient satisfaction and choise of prosthesis. Clin Oral Implants Res 2012; 32 (Suppl 6): 217–228
105. Abdou Elsyad M, Elgamal M, Mohammed Askar O, Youssef Al-Tonbary G: Patient satisfaction an oral health-related quality of life (OHRQoL) of conventional denture, fixed prosthesis and milled bar overdenture for All-on-4 implant rehabilitation. A crossover study. Clin Oral Implants Res 2019; 30: 1107–1117
106. Adell R, Eriksson B, Lekholm U, Brånemark PI, Jemt T: Long-term follow-up study of osseointegrated implants in the treatment of totally edentulous jaws. Int J Oral Maxillofac Implants 1990; 5(4): 347–59
107. Bakker MH, Vissink A, Meijer HJA, Ragoebar GM, Visser A: Mandibular implant-supported overdentures in (frail) elderly: A prospective study with 20-year follow-up. Clin Implant Dent Relat Res 2019; 21: 586–592
108. Passia N, Kern M: The single midline implant in the endentulous mandible: a systematic review. Clin Oral Investig 2014; 18: 1719–1724
109. Enami E, Alesawy A, de Grandmont P, Cerutti-Kopplin D, Kodama N, Menassa M, Rompré P, Durand R: A within s subject clinical trial on the conversion of mandibular two-implant to three-implant overdenture: Patient-centered outcomes and willingness to pay. Clin Oral Implants Res 2019; 30: 218–228
110. Wolfart S: Implantatprothetik – ein patientenorientiertes Konzept. Berlin: Quintessenz 2014
111. Rinke S, Fischer C: CAD/CAM gefertigte Stegkonstruktionen. Implantol 2012; 20: 65–74
112. Spiekermann H et al.: Farbatlanten der Zahnmedizin Bd. 10, Implantologie, Hrsg. Klaus H. Rateitschak und Herbert F. Wolf, Thieme Verlag Stuttgart, 1994
113. Emami E, Heydecke G, Rompré PH, de Grandmont P, Feine JS: Impact of implant support for mandibular dentures on satisfaction, oral and general health-related quality of life: a meta-analysis of randomized-controlled trials. Clin Oral Implants Res 2009 Jun; 20(6): 533–44
114. Schiegnitz E, Al-Nawas B: Narrow-diamter implants: A systematic review and meta-analysis. Clin Oral Implantts Res. 2018; 29(16): 21–40

115. Enkling N, Haueter M, Worni A, Müller F, Leles CR, Schimmel A: A prospective cohort study on survival and succes of one-piece mini-implants with associated changes in oral function: Five-year outcomes. Clin Oral Implants Res 2019; 30: 570–577
116. Balmer S, Mericske-Stern R: Implant-supported bridges in the edentulous jaw. Clinical aspects of a simple treatment concept, Schweiz Monatsschr Zahnmed, 2006, 116(7): 728–39
117. Maló P, de Araùjo Nobre M, Lopes A, Ferro A, Botto J: The All-on-4 concept for full-arch rehabilitation of the completely edentulous mandible: A longintudinal study with 10-18 years of follow-up. Clin Implant Dent Relat Res 2019; 21: 565–577
118. Gruber H, Solar P, Ulm C: Anatomie und atrophiebedingte Veränderungen der Kieferknochen, in: Watzek G: Enossale Implantate in der oralen Chirurgie, Quintessenz Berlin, 1993
119. Watson RM, David DM, Forman GH, Coward T: Considerations in design and fabrication of maxillary implant-supported prostheses. Int J Prosthodont 4, 1991: 232f
120. Kern JS, Wolfart S: S3-Leitlinie der DGZMK: Implantatprothetische Versorgung des zahnlosen Kiefers, 2020
121. Kern JS, Kern T, Wolfart S, Heussen N: A systematic review and meta-analysis of removable and fixed implant- supported prosthesesin edentulousjaws: post loading implant loss. Clin Oral Implants Res 2016; 27: 174–195
122. Wolfart S, Naujokat H, Wiltfang J, Kern M: Implantologie im zahnlosen Kiefer – Ein Update nach 25 Jahren. Implantologie 2017; 25(4): 327–344
123. Roccuzzo M , Bonino F, Guadioso L, Zwahlen M, Meijer HJ: What ist the optimal number of implants for removable reconstructions? A systematic review on implant-supported overdentures. Clin Oral Implants Res. 2012; 23 Suppl (6): 229–237
124. Mori G, Oda Y, Sakamoto K, Ito T, Yajima Y: Clinical evaluation of full-arch screw-retained implant supported fixed prostheses and full-arch telescopic-retained implant-supported fixed prostheses: A 5 -12 year follow-up retrospective study. Clin Oral Implants Res. 2019; 30: 197–205
125. Kern JS, Kern T, Wolfart S, Heussen N: A systematic review and meta-analysis of removable and fixed implant - supported prostheses in edentulousjaws: post loading implant loss. Clin Oral Implants Res 2016; 27: 174–195
126. Maló P, de Araùjo Nobre M, Lopes A, Ferro A, Nunes M: The All-on-4 concept for full-arch rehabilitation of the edentulous maxillae: A longitudinal study with 5-13 years of follow-up. Clin Implant Dent Relat Res 2019; 21: 538–549
127. Pieralli S, Kohal RJ, Rabel K, von Stein-Lausnitz M, Vach K, Spies BC: Clinical outcomes of partial and full-arch all ceramic implant-supported fixed dental prostheses. A systematic review and meta-analysis. Clin Oral Implants Res 2018; 29 Suppl 18: 224–236

Index